020839095 34

Ben

CW00693028

WHO'S HAVING YOUR BABY?

Beverley Lawrence Beech is the chair of the Association for Improvements in the Maternity Services and lay advisor to the National Perinatal Epidemiology Unit, Oxford. In 1982 she co-chaired a World Health Organisation conference in the United States on appropriate technology in antenatal care. In 1985 she chaired the campaign to reinstate Wendy Savage, the consultant obstetrician who was suspended for alleged professional incompetence and was subsequently exonerated. She also co-chaired a symposium at the Royal Society of Medicine on ultrasonography in obstetrics, and in 1987 she co-organised, with Janet Belaskas and Melody Weig, the first international conference on home birth.

She has contributed a chapter 'Know Your Rights: A Parents' Guide to Birth' in *Birth Matters*, edited by Ros Claxton (Unwin Paperbacks, 1986) and wrote a chapter on women's views of the birth process in *Benefits and Hazards of the New Obstetrics: Obstetrics for the 1990s*, edited by Professor Tim Chard and Dr Martin Richards (MacKeith Press, forthcoming).

As well as writing and campaigning on maternity issues, she regularly talks to childbirth, midwifery and medical groups in Britain. In 1989 she was invited to speak in Ireland, Italy and Germany.

She has two sons and lives in Buckinghamshire.

WHO'S HAVING YOUR BABY?

A HEALTH RIGHTS HANDBOOK FOR MATERNITY CARE

Beverley Lawrence Beech

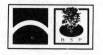

Bedford Square Press

Published by
BEDFORD SQUARE PRESS OF THE
National Council for Voluntary Organisations
26 Bedford Square, London WC1B 3HU

First published by Camden Press Ltd 1987
This edition published by Bedford Square Press 1991
© Beverley Lawrence Beech 1987, 1991

All rights reserved. No part of this publication may be reproduced or
transmitted, in any form or by any means, electronic, mechanical,
photocopying, recording or otherwise without the prior permission of the
publisher.

Typeset by AKM Associates (UK) Ltd, Southall, London
Printed and bound in Great Britain by J.W. Arrowsmith, Bristol
Cover printed by Heyford Press, Wellingborough

A catalogue record for this book is available from the British Library.

CONTENTS

FOREWORD

This book is written for women and families as an aid in helping them to get the maternity experience that they want. Sadly, it is not easy today for a woman and family to get the maternity experience that they prefer. During the last 10 years the Regional Office for Europe of the World Health Organisation has been carefully studying maternity services throughout the European region and evaluating the world scientific literature on this subject. This makes it abundantly clear that there has been a serious medicalisation of birth and birth services. In other words, pregnancy has been turned into an illness (which it is not) and birth has been turned into a surgical procedure (which it is not). Doctors and hospitals have unwittingly taken the control of the birth and what happens at the time of the birth away from the woman and her family. Pregnant and birthing women are told by health professionals what will happen to them and this is usually not negotiable. To question what the doctor or midwife says is to be a 'bad patient'. This bad patient will be immediately met with patronizing coersion. This of course is not always the case but it is the case often enough that the pregnant and birthing woman must be prepared for it. There are only a few places in Britain where a pregnant and birthing woman can get exactly the experiences she wants without some kind of struggle.

Part of the medicalisation of birth has been also been the use of more and more obstetrical interventions and technologies. Many of these technologies have never been adequately scientifically evaluated to determine whether or not they are really of any help. Consequently, one finds higher and higher rates of inappropriate use of obstetrical technologies and interventions in the European countries. A final result of the medicalisation and increasing use of various tests and machines is that the pregnant and birthing woman is no longer in control and no longer the centre of attention, but rather the doctor and the technology have become the stars. The fact that birth is one of the most important experiences in the life of the woman and the life of the family has been lost in the rush to assist.

All of the above problems with the evolution of maternity services are found in Britain, and in fact Britain was found by WHO studies to have higher rates of obstetrical interventions than any other country in Europe. What can the woman and the family in Britain do about this? When a woman finds herself pregnant how can she best find the kind of maternity service that she wishes and most importantly, how can the woman and the family get the maternity experience that they want? What the pregnant woman needs is the best possible information so that she can make the right choices. Fortunately in Britain there is the possibility for the woman to carefully read this book. This book will help the pregnant woman and her family to get the experience they want including not only the right kind of medical attention during pregnancy and birth, but also the various kinds of social and other benefits that are available during this crucial moment in life. I know of no other source of information better than this book for this purpose.

This book will also fully inform the pregnant woman and her family on their rights with regard to the services that are available. This is extremely important when dealing with the health care system as it is very difficult to learn your rights, whether it is in a clinic or the hospital. This also, incidentally, includes your rights if you are asked to be a research subject. This book clearly identifies these rights and gives assistance in ensuring that you can secure these rights.

This book will also help greatly to demystify the care that the pregnant and birthing woman receives. This is a very clear and very accurate description of all tests and procedures and this will dispel any notion that there is any magic in medical care. Furthermore, the information is given in a non-patronising way which is one of the biggest problems one faces in dealing with the health care system. The pros and cons and latest valid information on all procedures is clearly given. An excellent example of this is the balanced presentation of the value of ultrasound. Here all of the facts are given on both sides of the case and this allows the individual woman to then make the best possible informed choice about whether or not she wishes to have ultrasound.

In addition to assisting the individual woman and her family in getting the right maternity experience, this book also serves another

important function. Doctors and hospitals are attempting to look
out for the patient's best interest, but it is a reality that they are at
the same time looking out for their own interests. For this reason,
it is absolutely essential for people who use health care to be as
well organised as the providers of health care. Only in this way can
the consumers of health care ensure their own best interest in
using the health care system. I have known the author of this book
for over 10 years and watched her closely in all of her work. She is
the consummate consumer advocate. She gathers all the facts and
carefully evaluates them and can be absolutely relied upon with
her information. At the same time she knows how to deal with the
health care system and the health providers. This book carefully
tells women how they can organise themselves to advocate at the
local level for better care. The book even goes so far as to give you
examples of letters which can be used when contacting the various
parts of the health care system in demanding proper care. The
World Health Organisation strongly supports community participation and consumer rights in health care. This is an excellent
cookbook on how to accomplish this in the field of maternity
services in Britain.

The World Health Organisation believes that the most basic
requirement of good maternity services is the fully informed choice
of the woman using these services. The Regional Office for Europe
recently published a report 'Having a baby in Europe'. Let me
quote verbatim the last paragraph in this report which addresses
the essential place of informed choice in maternity care:

Each woman should have an informed choice concerning the
application of the care to herself. In recent times the concept
of 'informed consent' had become more accepted in health
care, but the word consent implies agreement to the choice
made by someone else. In hospitals today it is often the case
that the chief physician may decide that women may, for
example, walk around during labour if they choose. But
whatever the chief physician has not given explicit permission
to do is forbidden. This, of course, is not real choice. As stated
earlier, it is essential for the woman to feel she is in control if
she is to be able spontaneously and effectively to open herself
to give birth. Consequently, the feeling of having a choice and
thereby being in control is perhaps more important than what
is chosen. Everyone, including health providers, users and
society, agrees that the death of a woman or a baby is a tragedy
to be prevented if at all possible. At the same time, human
beings have always felt that certain other things are as important as survival, including the freedom to live their own lives

their own way and to make individual choices in line with
their own sense of values as well as the values of society.

This book is an outstanding source of full information for the
pregnant and birthing woman in Britain so that she can have true
informed choice.

In summary, this book is accurate, sensible and reliable. Too
often the health provider will tell a woman 'Trust me, I'm a doctor.'
I assure you that in fact what you can trust is this book. I would
wish that every country in the European region would have their
own version of this book. Every pregnant woman in Britain should
have a copy of this book and take it when going to the clinic or the
hospital.

Marsden G. Wagner
Responsible Officer, Maternal and Child Health
World Health Organisation

ACKNOWLEDGEMENTS

The first edition of this book has been written with the help and support of a great many people. Not least my two sons, David and Alan, who have tolerated my obsession with the word processor. It has also been written with the active and enthusiastic help of my colleagues, management, and volunteers of Health Rights. I would particularly like to thank the Association for Improvements in the Maternity Services for their help and support. A special thank you to Yvonne Baginski, Janette Brierley, Iain Chalmers, Mary Cronk, Carmel Fairmichael, Melanie Graham, Maddy Halliday, Mari Jenkins, Robin Lawson, Belinda Pratten, Jean Robinson, Christine Rodgers and Sandar Warshal for their enthusiasm and unfailing support, advice and wisdom, which many of them gave during the writing of this edition. Additionally, I would particularly like to thank Mary Renfrew for her time and the valuable suggestions she made on the new section on infant feeding, and to Marsden Wagner for his very generous foreword.

INTRODUCTION

Childbirth is one of the most momentous occasions in a woman's life, one she will remember with amazing clarity for decades afterwards.

It is only very recently that childbirth has moved from an intimate family occasion to an obstetric event, which takes place away from accustomed surroundings, in an atmosphere of haste and amongst an ever-changing collection of strangers.

Women rarely see childbirth before they themselves give birth, and as a result they have lost the knowledge of normality that our foremothers had.

The current issue in maternity care is 'choice'. Hospitals confidently publicise their wish to ensure that the parents have choice, but many of them keep very quiet about the way they ensure that very little choice is available, often making it extremely difficult for women to exercise that choice.

Martin Richards (a psychologist) illustrated perfectly the way in which choice is restricted by describing how a woman walked into her local supermarket and asked the manager what choice of fish was available, 'Well, we have whiting, herring, sole, plaice, mackerel, cod and rock salmon.' She said, 'How wonderful. Is it fresh fish?' 'No,' he replied. 'We only sell frozen.' The woman had a choice, either to go away empty handed or reluctantly accept some frozen fish. To her there had been no choice, but as far as the manager was concerned he had offered her a whole range. And so it is with many British hospitals. Many of them offer a wide range of medical procedures and drugs, but for women a normal birth (one that is allowed to take a psysiological course without interference from *routine* technological interventions), it may be quite difficult to arrange.

One of the results of this interest has been a blossoming of books on childbirth, with advice from every quarter and a multitude of leaflets. Whilst many of these books are helpful in some respects, the majority unfortunately fail to give women advice on how to make an informed decision about the care they want, or the questions they ought to be asking.

Many books and booklets are patronising in the extreme. A booklet published by the British Medical Association and the Royal Society of Medicine, 'You and Your Baby', states

> If he (the doctor) and a midwife are prepared to take the responsibility (for a home birth), then the NHS will make the best possible provision for your convenience and safety. If your doctor will not take this responsibility on himself, think very carefully before ignoring his advice. Remember that his concern is for your health and safety and that of your baby.

There is no suggestion that the doctor and midwife are there to *advise and support.* The booklet makes it quite clear that one should not make a move without first consulting the doctor. Such attitudes reduce women to the level of children: 'do as you are told because doctor knows best'. Such books ignore the fact that all but a very few mothers are adults, and that they will have the responsibility of nurturing, caring and loving their new baby, and fail to recognise that a great deal of routine procedures used in maternity care have little scientific evidence to support their use. In other words, there are many occasions when doctors and midwives do not know best. It is time that the mother's role was recognised as one of the most responsible jobs anyone can do. This responsibility should be respected, not diminished by treating pregnant women as passive, infantile, baby carriers.

For women who want to go into hospital and leave the decisions about their care to the 'experts', there is plenty of choice and little difficulty in getting it. But those who want a normal or 'natural' birth have a much harder time getting what they want. They are often dependent on the good will of the midwives to help them. If the midwife doesn't recognise that what she is offering is a distortion of normal childbirth, then the woman will be unlikely to give birth in the way she wants unless she has the information to help her make the right decisions for herself. For many women childbirth is a lottery: a woman has to rely on the chance that she may be allocated to a midwife who really wants to encourage a normal birth and do all she can to help the woman achieve it.

Current obstetric mythology suggests that maternity care is fashioned to respond to women's needs. In many hospitals women are being given 'birth plans' to ensure that they record the choices they have made. This gives the hospital the opportunity to demonstrate that they take the mother's decisions seriously by putting the plan in her case notes. The reality is often very different: the majority of British women will not have a 'natural' birth, particularly if they are first-time mothers. They will invariably be persuaded to agree to interventions, and many of those interventions are carried out routinely with little thought for the needs of individual mothers and babies. Many of these interventions pervert the 'normality' of labour.

There are frequent discussions about what is a 'natural/normal' birth. It is generally accepted that it is a birth that follows a normal physiological path without needing obstetric interventions such as electronic foetal monitoring, induction or acceleration, epidural anaesthesia, forceps delivery, vacuum extraction or caesarean section. Yet, apart from the last three interventions, all the former will qualify for an entry on your case notes as 'normal delivery'.

So, it is possible for Mrs Smith to be admitted and have her pubic hair partially shaved. She may then have her waters broken, a foetal scalp electrode attached, a drip set up and, because of the disruption to the normal process of labour and the increased pain, she may then be offered drugs or an epidural. If she is lucky she will give birth without a forceps delivery and then find that her case notes state that she has had a 'normal delivery'. It is time that we stopped referring to such births as normal, they are vaginal deliveries. A birth cannot be normal if a woman has a drip set up, electronic foetal monitoring, a foetal scalp electrode attached, and epidural anaesthesia as all these procedures can pervert the course of a normal labour.

It is all very well knowing that an induction is a method of making the uterus contract and labour start, but what use is this if one knows nothing about the risks of the procedure and how it affects the normal process of birth? Unfortunately, very few childbirth books actually discuss these issues; they have drawings and diagrams of the equipment, but do not give the women sufficient information about the implications of such interventions so they can consider, on an informed basis, whether to have an induction or acceleration or not.

According to the World Health Organisation report 'Having a Baby in Europe', Britain has one of the highest levels of obstetric interventions when compared with other European countries for which data are available.

How is it that many technological interventions are used and yet women still expect, or are told that they are having, a normal birth? Unfortunately, because they are not provided with the information, very few women understand that the majority of obstetric interventions run the risk of perverting normal labour, and many doctors and midwives have become so used to carrying out these procedures they often fail to think about the implications for individual women and babies.

During the 1960s it was common for women to have interventions (like breaking the waters) as a matter of course, and if they questioned it they were told, in no uncertain terms, that this is the hospital policy and that was that. Since that time, and mainly due to the activities of the Association for Improvements in the Maternity Services (AIMS), the legality of giving treatment to a woman without her consent, and often directly against her expressed wishes, has been challenged. Attitudes changed, almost overnight, and midwives and doctors have learned to be 'nice'. They have taken on public relations in a big way, and it has made it very much more difficult for women to argue.

In the bad old days, a bossy domineering midwife or doctor was easy to identify and easier to oppose – at least you knew exactly who the enemy was. Now it was a much greater problem. One of the most difficult things for a first-time mother is to arm herself adequately to deal with the emotional and subtle pressures that may well be put on her to agree with routine obstetric interventions.

Women are still getting unncessary treatment and interventions, but many of them have been persuaded to accept it. The tactic is quite easy. First the midwife arrives and announces that she is going to break the waters and a doctor will come and attach a foetal scalp electrode. The mother says that she would rather not have that because she has heard that the technique is not very effective and, furthermore, increases the baby's breathing rate (a possible indication that the baby is feeling pain). The midwife then responds with a serious look and a benign smile. 'Well, of course, Mrs Smith, I respect your wish not to have foetal monitoring, but I do feel I should draw your attention to the fact that babies sometimes become distressed in labour and that can happen very quickly. When it does happen the brain can be deprived of oxygen and if that were to happen for any length of time then you could have a brain-damaged baby. Or worse, the baby could die. Of course, the decision is yours, but I must warn you that you will have to take full responsibility for your decision, which will be against medical advice. And, of course, I do have the best interests of your baby at heart, we never do anything routinely at this hospital.' Big smile and a classic example of shroud waving.

Very few women threatened with the damage or death of their

baby are going to do anything other than give in to such tactics, unless they understand the risks of electronic foetal monitoring and know what questions they ought to be asking. For a first-time mother it is a tactic that is almost impossible to counter and many, many women give in.

This book has been written as a first step towards informing women, to help them understand the issues better and what real choices there are.

In many British hospitals today, particularly teaching hospitals and consultant units, there is very little real choice. Women are required to fit into the obstetric care that is considered to be best for them, despite research evidence showing that obstetric and teaching hospitals and private maternity units are the most dangerous places of all. There is little question of women deciding what they want and the midwifery service taking note and doing its best to fulfill these demands. Few women have continuity of care and the likelihood of them getting the kind of birth they want depends to a great extent on a form of lottery. If they are lucky they will be attended by midwives who will do all they can to ensure that the birth is as normal as possible and the technology and drugs are only used when needed and in appropriate circumstances. Finding these midwives in a large hospital depends to a great extent on the luck of the draw. The fragmented care on offer in so many large hospitals will only change when midwives begin to take over full responsibility for all women, work in teams, and give full continuity of care.

Midwives are the most qualified professionals to deal with normal childbirth, yet over the years their jobs have been fragmented and women have been forced into accepting a standard of care that shunts them through as if on a conveyor belt. Until there is a return to good midwifery practice, in which midwives reclaim their role as 'with-women' and all women know that during their pregnancy and labours they will be cared for by a midwife they have known for the last nine months, little is going to be done about improving maternity care. The Association of Radical Midwives in a booklet called *The Vision* has proposed a restructuring of midwifery so that women have continuity of care and actually know their attendants well. The sooner these proposals are implemented the better.

Until these changes are made, women will have to fight and argue for what they want. They take part in a lottery, with the lucky ones finding a midwife who responds to their needs and does all she can to ensure a normal birth. For those women who have the additional burden of not speaking English, not having adequate translation facilities, and often having to deal with the institutional and individual racism in the NHS, the struggle to obtain the kind of care they want is even more difficult. Those women who book a home birth, a domino delivery or a GP unit birth, stand a much greater chance of getting what they want because, in the main, midwives working with this kind of care are more responsive to the needs of individual women, and not so pressured to obey the dictats of 'hospital policy'.

Booking a home birth, a domino delivery or a GP unit birth is not easy, except in one or two exceptional areas. You only have to examine the statistics by health authority to see very clearly that home and domino births hardly exist, and GP units are being closed with frightening rapidity. There are many who believe that this is a direct result of vigorous opposition by obstetricians who are more concerned with extending their influence and control than they are in ensuring the safest possible delivery for the mother and baby.

This book has been written to help you get what you want. It will not guarantee that you get the kind of birth you wish but it may well increase your chances.

1

THE CHOICE OF ANTENATAL CARE

> We unhesitatingly accept the often reiterated claim of antenatal care as a means of reducing perinatal and neonatal mortality, what exactly antenatal care consists of and how it works has been less clear to us (The Report of the Social Services Committee on Perinatal and Neonatal Mortality, 1980 (The Short Report).

Antenatal care was first introduced around 1915. At that time there was concern about Britain having higher mortality rates than other countries (much the same anxieties were expressed in the Short Report), and like the Short Report no evidence was presented to show that antenatal care would achieve a reduction in mortality or morbidity. By 1932 40 per cent of women received antenatal care, by 1937 this had risen to 54 per cent. Today, over 90 per cent of women receive antenatal care.

Initially antenatal care was provided on the basis of educating mothers to take care of themselves and their babies; after the First World War that emphasis changed to one of supervision of pregnant women by professionals.

A great deal of attention is focused on 'treating and monitoring' women in antenatal clinics, yet little has been done to address the social needs of many women.

If you live in a damp, overcrowded, two-roomed flat with an unemployed husband and a couple of small children you are unlikely to have a good standard of health. The everyday stresses in your life are likely to be considerable and it is hardly surprising that many women living in these circumstances smoke cigarettes. It is interesting to note that instead of concentrating on improving these conditions, campaigns are mounted to stop women smoking (usually by making them feel guilty). The authorities do not address the question of *why* women started smoking in the first place and why they still continue.

The health problems of many families will not be 'cured' by getting women into antenatal clinics and monitoring them. It will have to be dealt with by a commitment to improve the quality of their lives and particularly their housing and social conditions. The World Health Organisation is already addressing this enormous problem with their 'Health For All' targets. The UK is a signatory to the WHO Health 2000 Targets, yet it is slow to take action, despite its poor health record compared to many other developed countries.

Modern antenatal care offers women a series of checks in order to establish the state of their health and that of their baby and, hopefully, detect any problems. For example, by routinely testing the woman's urine it is possible to detect and treat infections one of which, pyelonephritis, can have very serious implications for the mother and baby.

Unfortunately, the quality of antenatal care around the country is very variable and too many antenatal clinics are overcrowded. Women often find they have little time to discuss their care with the professionals involved, and often are required to sit patiently for many hours before being seen for a few minutes by harassed staff. Ann Oakley commented, following her review of antenatal care, that the question is not 'Why do some women fail to attend for antenantal care by why do women *attend* antenatal clinics?'

There are studies which demonstrate the benefits of antenatal care can cause problems. A study in Aberdeen of women receiving routine antenatal care showed that many women were overdiagnosed as having pre-eclampsia, high blood pressure, or small-for-gestational-age babies (Hall, 1987). Such over-diagnosis can lead to over-investigation, unnecessary admission to hospital and induction or operative delivery, with all the attendant risks, trauma and upset that this may cause. At the same time the study found that the majority of justified antenatal admissions were emergencies and could not have been predicted by antenatal care.

Before you decide which type of care you want you should check out the antenatal clinics to see what they are like. Modern antenatal clinics are often overcrowded, and many women expect to wait many hours for a brief and cursory examination.

Because of inadequate funding of the National Health Service many women are finding it increasingly difficult to find the kind of antenatal care they want. They are herded into clinics to wait patiently to see a doctor or midwife they have not seen before and in all probability will not see again.

Check that each woman has an individual appointment time, find out from other women how long they generally wait. If you find that a dozen or so women all have the same appointment time or that it is common to wait anything over an hour, then find yourself another antenatal clinic or consider having antenatal care in your area or own home. As long ago as 1954 the DHSS issued a circular stating that the system of giving large numbers of women the same appointment times (block booking) should stop (HM (54) 52). We are still patiently waiting for the Health Authorities and Health Boards to take notice of this circular.

When you attend an antenatal clinic you will be weighed, have a blood sample taken, asked to give a sample of urine, and examined to check that you are fit and well.

It is generally accepted that a woman is checked:

- every four weeks until she is 28 weeks pregnant, then
- every two weeks until she is 36 weeks pregnant and then
- every week until the baby is born

These rules are not based on any kind of scientific study or evaluation. They evolved over a period of time and it became generally accepted as 'a good thing'. The Aberdeen study, however, showed that there is little reason for fit and healthy low-risk women to attend antenantal clinics up to 32 weeks and concluded that it would be better for the routine checks to be carried out by the midwives in the women's own homes or in local clinics.

In some areas, therefore, providing you are fit and healthy, the midwife, or doctor, may decide that they do not wish to see you quite so often. Equally, they may feel that they wish to see you more often, particularly if you have a problem that they want to keep an eye on. If you find that in between appointments you wish to see them, you can telephone and discuss the matter and arrange an appointment.

Women concerned that they may be at increased risk of carrying an abnormal baby and want to be checked will need to sign on for antenatal care as early as possible, so that they can have whatever screening tests are appropriate. Some of these tests (e.g. chorionic villus sampling) are carried out early in pregnancy (around nine to ten weeks).

In good antenatal clinics you will have plenty of time to discuss the kind of care you want and to put any questions you want to ask. If you do not know why you are being given a specific test, or the reasons for the questions they are asking, you should speak up. Don't be afraid to say, 'I don't understand, will you please explain that again.' Very often the staff will use jargon which will be meaningless to you. You are not being silly if you ask them to explain, or ask them about a problem that has been worrying you – that is what they are there for. They have been dealing with pregnant women for a long time but this may be your first baby and you may have a lot of questions you want answered.

Sometimes the staff make it quite clear that they think your question is stupid or they answer in such a way that you are still none the wiser. Don't put up with it: it is your body and your baby and you have every right to an explanation. If you have not understood what they have said, or they have tried to avoid answering your question, then ask again. You can always say 'Thank you for that information but you have not answered my question. What I asked was . . .' and repeat the original question. That usually brings forth a more sensible response. If it does not, then say it again.

If you find yourself sitting for hours on end in a busy antenatal clinic why not get together and persuade the women present to send their own letter of protest to the Health Authority? If you complain on your own the Health Authority can easily dismiss you as a 'complainer', if, however, large numbers of women are also complaining, the Health Authority and Health Districts will be forced into taking action. They will not be able to ignore a mass complaint. It is because women are reluctant to complain collectively about hospitals with poor standards that the care does not improve. Those who shout loudest usually get the attention. Unfortunately, pregnant women very rarely shout and that is why the care in some areas is as bad as it is.

You may find that you can no longer accept the care that is being offered in the clinic of your choice. In that case you can arrange alternative antenatal care by writing to the Supervisor of Midwives, along the following lines:

Dear . . .
I have been attending . . . . . antenatal clinic since . . . . . (insert date). I regret to say that I rarely wait less than . . . hours/ minutes to be seen and when I am it is rarely by the same person as last time.

I am not prepared to accept this standard of care and therefore I do not intend returning for any more antenatal appointments at this clinic. I am concerned to ensure that I receive the necessary antenatal care and I would appreciate it, therefore, if you would make arrangements for me to be seen, by a midwife, either in my own home or at my local GP's surgery.

Yours sincerely

This letter should be addressed to the Supervisor of Midwives at the hospital you are attending.

You could then contact your local Community Health Council (CHC) (in Scotland these are called Local Health Councils and in Northern Ireland they are called District Committees) and ask them to take up this issue. Send a copy of your letter to the chairs of the Regional Health Authority (Scotland: Regional Health Board; Northern Ireland; Health and Social Services Board) and District Health Authority (Scotland: Health Districts; Northern Ireland: Health and Social Services District), your MP and the local press. You can find their addresses in your local library or CHC offices. In this way everyone will know that the clinic is not up to standard and may begin to do something about it.

You may be told that there are insufficient staff to deal with such a request and that they do not provide this service. You could then remind them that they have a statutory obligation to provide maternity care and you have no intention of attending a clinic which, in your view, provides sub-standard care.

TYPE OF BOOKING

The type of antenatal care you receive is often linked to the kind of birth you choose (see chapters 5 and 6). So you have to make these decisions at the same time, otherwise you may find yourself wanting, for example, to have your baby in a consultant unit, while preferring to have your antenatal care locally. Not all Health Authorities and Health Boards provide a wide selection of alternatives and it is better to sort out what is on offer in your area, and what you want, before you commit yourself.

For many women the first step is taken when she arrives at the GP's surgery saying that she is pregnant. The doctor will confirm the pregnancy and then say 'I will book you into the . . . maternity unit.' What s/he rarely says is 'Mrs Smith, where would you like to give birth?' S/he is not likely to tell the woman that she has a choice:

Type of booking	Possible varieties of antenatal care
GP unit birth	Local GP's surgery or midwives' clinic
Consultant unit birth	Hospital antenatal clinic
Shared-care birth	Hospital antenatal clinic
	Local GP's clinic or midwives' clinic
	At home
Domino delivery	Local GP's surgery or midwives' clinic
	At home
Home birth	At home
	Local GP or midwives' clinic

If you want a type of care that is not available in your area you will have to decide whether or not you are going to argue and insist that it is provided. If you decide to do so, be sure that you contact Health Rights if you are in London, or AIMS or other childbirth organisations for support and help. Many pregnant women find it very stressful to argue unsupported and alone.

The GPs and midwives ought to tell you what the options are, but in many areas they do not – often taking the easy route and booking women automatically into the nearest consultant unit.

Once you have signed an FP24 (Family Health Services Authority (FHSA) 24 Form, in Scotland Form D10) for maternity care with your GP s/he cannot strike you off her/his list, without your consent or the consent of the FHSA (in Scotland this role is taken by the Secretary of State for Scotland and the Health Board). S/he is also responsible for finding you a suitable place to give birth to your baby. If, therefore, you are having problems booking into a particular hospital, it is the GP's responsibility to find a solution which is acceptable to you.

There are various types of antenatal care from which you can choose:

Shared care

Antenatal care is shared between your midwife and/or doctor and hospital. If your own doctor does not offer this service, you can, for the period of your pregnancy, change to another doctor who does. Look at the list of local doctors, available from your local library, post office or local Community Health Council (Scotland: Local Health Councils; Northern Ireland: District Committees) and contact those with 'GPO' (General Practitioner Obstetrician) after their name (they do the obstetric care); or ask your doctor to recommend a General Practitioner (GP) who does provide shared care, telephone your local National Childbirth Trust (NCT) branch or ask local women.

Local GP units

In some areas you may be fortunate enough to have a local GP unit, but they are often under threat of closure as a means of saving money.

With a GP unit you have a greater chance of continuity of care throughout pregnancy and birth, but it is important to check that the GP unit functions independently from the hospital. Some consultants lay down rules for the GPs, particularly where the unit is part of the consultant's unit, and the GPs and midwives are often required to follow hospital policy.

Some hospitals provide separate rooms or equipment for the GPs and local midwives to use which are integrated into the consultant unit. Some units simply have a number of beds which are designated as 'GP beds', a very unsatisfactory system since there is no identifiable demarcation between the GP 'unit' and the rest of the hospital.

Total care from the hospital

This means visiting the hospital for all care including all antenatal care. This kind of care is inappropriate for the majority of fit and healthy women, it is not even appropriate for many high-risk women (these are women who have been defined by the hospital as either having problems during their pregnancy or who are perceived as likely to have problems during pregnancy or labour), many of whom would benefit from continuity of community care (seeing the same people locally at each antenatal visit). For example, a woman with high blood pressure may feel better having care locally, with the occasional visit to the hospital, than making frequent hospital visits, which may in themselves create stress from the greater amount of travelling and long waits at busy antenatal clinics.

Some hospitals have recognised the advantages of giving high-risk women continuity of care within the hospital and have provided facilities. The John Radcliffe Hospital in Oxford has provided just such a clinic for high-risk women and this has been very much welcomed by the women who attend.

If you are defined as high-risk you should find our precisely why. Check with a community midwife or one of the childbirth groups. It is possible for the majority of high-risk women to receive their ante-natal care locally, if that is what they want.

Antenatal clinics in the community

Some hospital doctors hold antenatal clinics in local health clinics or the surgery of a group practice. Check whether or not there are any in your area.

Home birth

With most home births the midwife will give you antenatal care in your own home, or at the local GP/midwives' clinic.

YOUR RIGHTS

The fundamental principle of which many women are unaware is that it is *your body and your baby* and the staff do not have the right to carry out any treatment without your consent. Obviously if there is an emergency of some kind then the staff could act; but such emergencies are very rare and staff would have to be very sure of the necessity of what they are doing before going ahead, or they could find themselves facing a legal action for assault.

Many women are told that, for example, 'You have to have an ultrasound'. You do not. If you do not want it you do not have to accept it. Whether or not it is hospital policy to screen everyone is irrelevant. If you do not want a particular treatment you have every right to say 'Thank you very much, but I have decided not to take your advice'. Unfortunately, far too many professionals have forgotten that ultimately they are paid by you and me (through taxation) and they are there to provide a service. They are not there to force women into accepting whatever *they* deem to be appropriate. If you find yourself at odds with the staff on such issues contact AIMS immediately, or Health Rights if you are in London. You should not argue alone, unless you are very sure of your grounds. Pregnant women can feel very vulnerable and prefer to have someone assist them (either their parter or someone from the user groups).

Once you have signed on with your GP for maternity care s/he does not have the right to strike you off without applying to the FHSA (in Scotland the equivalent of an FHSA is the Primary Care Division of the Regional Health Board; in Northern Ireland, Central Services Agency) for permission to do so. Should s/he strike you off without your consent, or before applying to the FHSA for permission, you can make a formal complaint to the FHSA stating that s/he has broken her/his contract.

You do not *have* to see a GP. You can apply directly to the Supervisor of Midwives at your local maternity unit for antenatal care from the midwives only.

You have the right to sign on for maternity care with a GP other than the one with whom you are registered. This means that if you are ill with a condition not related to pregnancy (eg. 'flu) then you see you own GP. It should be noted, however, that many GPs resent their patients signing on with another GP for maternity care and strike them off their list (sometimes they strike off the whole family).

Morally, your partner, friend or relative has every right to be with you at antenatal appointments, although they have no *legal* right to be there at all. If you wish him/her to be there you can simply refuse to co-operate unless s/he stays. Threatening to leave often produces the desired result.

Just because you have made a booking for a specific type of care it does not mean that you are compelled to continue with it from then on. If you are not satisfied, find out what the alternatives are and change. If there is any argument, contact the user groups and approach the local Community Health Council for help.

If you find that you are not happy with your antenatal care then you have the right to change the arrangements. If you have booked with:

The consultant. Write to, or see, your GP and ask him/her to change the booking to another consultant or ask for shared GP/ midwifery care or midwifery care only. In the latter case, write directly to the Supervisor of Midwives and tell her that you are cancelling your booking with your consultant and wish to have midwifery care only.

The GP. Write to the Supervisor of Midwives and ask for midwifery care only; write to the Family Health Services Authority (Scotland: Primary Care Division of the Regional Health Board; Northern Ireland: Central Services Agency) and ask them to allocate another GP.

The midwife. Write to the Supervisor of Midwives and state that you are no longer prepared to be attended by midwife X and ask for another midwife to be allocated. You have the right to refuse to see a particular midwife at any time.

Some women have been told that they cannot have antenatal care until they have booked into hospital, or found a GP to cover for a home birth. No woman should become involved with finding a GP to cover a home birth (see the Home Birth Chapter 5), write immediately to the Supervisor of Midwives and ask her to provide a midwife for a home birth. Point out that you have not yet received antenatal care, despite Government and Health Authority suggestions that all women should book for antenatal care as soon as possible.

Some obstetricians refuse to do special tests ordered by the midwife, and insist that she refers you via a GP. A midwife has the right to refer you for special tests if you both feel that they are necessary. Any obstetrician refusing to act on the midwife's referral should be reported to the District General Manager immediately and the Supervisor of Midwives should be asked to support the midwife's action.

2

MATERNITY BENEFITS

DENTAL TREATMENT

You have a right to free NHS dental treatment if you are pregnant and were pregnant when the dentist accepted you for treatment, and for a year after your baby's birth. A leaflet D11 – NHS Dental Treatment will give you more information. It is available from CHCs, libraries and Social Security offices.

FREE PRESCRIPTIONS

You have a right to free NHS prescriptions while you are pregnant and for a year after your baby's birth.

You can apply by completing a form FW8 as soon as you are sure that you are pregnant. If you are claiming for free prescriptions after the baby is born then ask for a form P11. These forms can be obtained from your GP, midwife or health visitor or Social Security office.

If you want to claim a refund for a prescription you have already paid for you must claim within *one month*. Ask the chemist for a receipt form FP57 (EC57 in Scotland).

FREE MILK AND VITAMINS

If you are receiving Income Support you are entitled to tokens which can be exchanged for 7 pints or 8 half-litres of cows' milk each week for each of your children under five. You can use the tokens to get 900g of dried milk each week at maternity clinics and child health clinics for each of your babies under one year old.

If you become pregnant you should tell your social security

office and let them know the date your baby is due, so that you can get tokens for 7 pints or 8 half-litres of milk each week for yourself until your baby is born.

If you're a mother or expectant mother you can get free vitamins for yourself while you are pregnant or breast-feeding, and for your children aged under five. Ask for them at a maternity clinic or child health clinic and show your Income Support payment book or, if you're paid by girocheque, the letter that came with the girocheque.

If you are getting Family Credit and have children under five years of age you cannot get free milk, apparently the rates of Family Credit were increased because of this.

If you have got babies under one year you can get dried milk for them at specially reduced prices at maternity clinics and child health clinics. Show your Family Credit order book or, if you're paid by direct credit into your bank or building society account, the letter that notified you of the award of benefit.

TRAVELLING EXPENSES

If you are getting Income Support or Family Credit you can claim your fares to and from hospital. See leaflet H11 NHS hospital travel costs.

If you have a low income it is possible that you are entitled to claim your travelling expenses for your journeys to antenatal clinics and other hospital appointments. Close relatives, who are also on a low income, can also claim their fares when they visit you in hospital. Ask the midwives at the clinic, or ask to see the hospital social worker. Claim on Form H11 which you can get from your Social Security office or post office.

TIME OFF TO ATTEND ANTENATAL CLINICS

Your employer must pay you for time off while you keep appointments for antenatal care. Some employers may require proof that you have attended the clinics, showing them your 'co-operation' card is sufficient proof. A 'co-operation card' is a small card which you will be given at your first antenatal appointment. It has a record of your blood pressure, results of urine tests and other brief details of your pregnancy. Pregnant women are asked to carry it with them during their pregnancy.

STATUTORY MATERNITY PAY

Statutory Maternity Pay (SMP) is a new maternity scheme which will be operated by your employer. It replaces the old style maternity allowance and maternity pay. Like maternity pay, you do not have to plan to return to work to get it.

You can get SMP if *both* the following apply:

- You have been in the same employment for at least six months by the 15th week *before the baby is due*. (Ask your employers if you are not sure you have worked there long enough, or contact the Maternity Alliance or an advice agency). You are still in the job in this 15th week. (It does not matter if you are off work sick, or on holiday).
- Your average weekly earnings is over £46 per week.

If you are not sure if you are entitled to SMP, ask anyway. Your employers will work out whether or not you should get it.

You may also be able to get SMP if, because of your pregnancy, you were dismissed before the 26th week, or if your baby was born early.

SMP can be paid for up to 18 weeks. Payment will be made for any 18-week period between week 11 before the birth and week 11 after the birth. Week 11 before the birth is the earliest you can get SMP. It will not be paid if your baby is stillborn before this.

Statutory Maternity Pay (SMP) is a weekly payment, but your employer will usually pay you at the time you would have received your normal wages.

There are two rates of SMP. If you have been in the same employment for at least two years, by the 15th week before the baby is due, for at least 16 hours a week; or part-time for five years for at least 8 hours a week, you can get a higher rate of SMP, which is 90 per cent of your normal wages for the first six weeks of your SMP. After that you will get the lower rate, which is £39.25 for the remainder of your SMP period. If you have been in the same employment for between 26 weeks and two years, by the 15th week before the baby is due, you will get the lower rate throughout the SMP period.

You can apply for SMP by telling your employer that you intend to stop work because of your pregnancy. You must do this at least three weeks before the date you intend to stop work.

Women who have two or more jobs are entitled to SMP for each job. Where her earnings are below the lower earnings limit (of £46) for each contract, her earnings can be aggregated to bring her above the level. In this case, SMP will be appropriated between employers.

Some of the snags

- A woman must have reached the 11th week before confinement or have given birth prematurely.

- You must give medical evidence of your pregnancy, usually form Mat B1. Failure to give this evidence or the necessary notice can be a reason to refuse to pay SMP.
- You may have to pay tax and National Insurance contributions on SMP.
- If you work for an agency you may not be able to claim if there has been a break in your contracts between agencies during the qualifying period.
- The rules entitle you to leave work from the 14th week before the estimated date of confinement. If, however, you leave before the 11th week then you forfeit you right to return to work.

Further information

The Maternity Alliance has published a leaflet 'Pregnant at Work' which will give you further information.

You can obtain more details by asking for a leaflet NI17A – Maternity Benefits from your Social Security office.

MATERNITY ALLOWANCE

For those mothers who can't get SMP but have recently given up their job, or changed jobs, or have recently been self-employed, or did not give three weeks notice before they stopped work, may be able to get up to 18 weeks Maternity Allowance (£35.70 a week) from the Department of Social Security (DSS).

To qualify you must have paid full rate NI contributions for at least 26 of of the 52 weeks ending with the 15th week before the week in which your baby is due.

The payment period for Maternity Allowance starts 11 weeks before your baby is due. But if you are still employed at the time your Maternity Allowance may start later. Payment will normally be made for a 'core period' of 13 weeks beginning six weeks before your baby is due, but it is up to you to decide when to take the remaining five weeks. You can take some before and some after, or all before or all after. But you cannot get the Allowance for any week in which you are working.

You can claim this allowance by obtaining a form MA1 from the Social Security officer or antenatal clinic. You should send the form to your Social Security office after you are 26 weeks pregnant. Be sure you send your maternity certificate (form MatB1) from your doctor or midwife (and keep a record, in a safe place, of the date you sent this form off – you will then be in a confident position to argue should the form have 'gone astray').

If you have already applied for Statutory Maternity Pay from your employer s/he will normally keep your maternity certificate but you can ask for it back so that you can make this claim.

If your employer has refused to pay you SMP s/he should issue you with a form SMP1 which you should send with your claim for Maternity Allowance.

It is very important that you do not delay in sending in your application. If you leave it too late you may not get part of your allowance.

If are already off work and getting Statutory Sick Pay this will stop when you change to SMP or Maternity Allowance. (You are not allowed to be sick *and* pregnant!) You still have to tell your employer three weeks before you stop work because of your pregnancy.

MATERNITY PAYMENT FROM THE SOCIAL FUND

If you or your partner are getting Income Support or Family Credit you may be able to have a Maternity Payment from the new Social Fund to help pay for things for your new baby.

If you are adopting a baby you can apply for a payment if the baby is not more than 12 months old when you apply. (Clearly officialdom believes that babies over 12 months old don't need clothes or equipment!) You can apply at any time from when you adopt to up to three months afterwards.

The payment is £100 for each baby expected or born, but the total amount will be reduced by any savings over £500 that you, or your partner or any dependent children who live with you have. For every £1 of savings over £500, £1 will be deducted.

If you want to apply for a Social Fund Maternity Payment you should write to your Social Security office for a claim form, SF100. You should send your maternity certificate (form MatB1) with this application, but if you do not have it then you can send in a copy of your antenatal clinic card instead. *You can apply until your baby is three months old.* If you are claiming after the birth send a copy of your baby's birth certificate instead of MatB1.

CHILD BENEFIT

If you have been living in Britain for at least six months you can claim Child Benefit. It is paid by a booklet of orders which you can cash at the post office each week or once a month. Mothers under sixteen are also able to claim.

The Benefit is £7.25 a week for each child and you can claim it by getting a claim form, address label CH3 and leaflet CH1, from your Social Security office.

If you receive Supplementary Benefit the Social Security office will deduct Child Benefit (and One-Parent Benefit) when you claim for the dependent child.

ONE-PARENT BENEFIT

If you have been living in Britain for at least six months and you are a single parent you can claim this benefit, which is £5.60 per week. Mothers under 16 can also claim.

You should ask at the Social Security office for a leaflet CH11.

HOUSING BENEFIT

If you have difficulty paying your rent and poll tax (Community Charge) then you may be eligible for Housing Benefit. If you are on Income Support or have an income below a certain level then you may be entitled. You cannot get Housing Benefit if your savings are more than £8,000, and it can be reduced if you have more than £3,000 in savings. The system is very complicated so you should seek advice from a housing office, advice centre or Citizens Advice Bureau. Your Housing Benefit may also increase after your baby is born, so don't forget to tell the Local Authority.

STILLBIRTH OR MISCARRIAGE

The death of a baby is a traumatic and distressing event leaving many parents unaware that they still have entitlements to a number of benefits. If you miscarry after the twenty-eighth week of pregnancy, or your baby is stillborn your entitlement to benefits does not change. The doctor or midwife will give you a certificate of stillbirth which you should give to the register of Births and Deaths (at your Town Hall). If no doctor or midwife was present at the birth, ask the registrar for Form 35, fill it in and give it back to the registrar. The registrar will give you a certificate of burial.

YOUR RIGHTS

The rules and regulations surrounding maternity benefits are often extremely complex, not helped by the authorities' reluctance to promote and comply with the regulations. If you are not sure about your entitlement then contact the Maternity Allowance Alliance, 15 Britannia Street, London WC1X 9JP. They have produced two very helpful leaflets 'Money for Mothers and Babies' and 'Pregnant at Work', which are also available in Bengali as well as Cantonese. The leaflets are free but please send an sae. The Maternity Alliance has also produced a very useful book about parents' rights at work – *Working Parents' Rights*.

3

ANTENATAL SCREENING

The purpose of antenatal care is to identify any woman who has problems during pregnancy and any baby who may have congential defects or conditions which could affect its future health.

The vast majority of babies are fit and healthy and babies with such problems are rare. While the purpose of antenatal screening is to detect potential problems, little research has been done to establish how much added stress healthy mothers suffer as a result of this constant harping on problems they 'might' have. The following is a list of the tests which are available, some routinely, some done only when there are indications that there may be problems. The tests have been listed in roughly the order in which you may come across them, with some of the more uncommon tests at the end.

Test	To detect
Blood pressure	That your blood pressure is not rising or falling too much
Urine	Bacteria, glucose, oestriol, protein
Blood tests	Identification of blood type
	Rhesus factor and antibodies
	Rubella antibodies
	Alpha foeto-proteins
	Placental lactogen
	AIDS (in some areas)
	Syphilis, gonorrhea and some other sexually transmitted diseases

Chorionic Villus sampling	It detects the same things as amniocentesis but does *not* detect spina bifida
Electronic foetal heart monitoring	The baby's heartbeat
Foetal movement counting	A baby which may be becoming distressed

Amniocentesis	Neural tube defects
	  Anencephaly
	  Spina bifida
	Down's syndrome and some other chromosome disorders
	Some inherited diseases
	Sex prediction

Ultrasound	Establish the estimated date of delivery Neural tube defects Detecting twins, triplets, etc. Small-for-dates babies
X-rays	To determine pelvic shape and size of the mother (after the 32nd week)

The following descriptions of these tests are in alphabetical order.

AMNIOCENTESIS

The amniocentesis test is most often done to detect chromosome disorders of which Down's syndrome and spina bifida are the most common. It will also detect some very rare inherited diseases and it will also identify the sex of the baby.

It is usually carried out as an outpatient test and can be done in a morning or afternoon appointment. You do not have to be admitted to hospital.

An ultrasound scan will be done to make sure that you are sixteen weeks pregnant and to check the position of the baby and the placenta. You need a full bladder for this scan.

Your skin will be cleaned with antiseptic, and a small injection may be given to numb the area. A fine needle is then passed through your abdomen into the womb, and a sample (about four teaspoonsful) of the fluid that surrounds the baby is removed with a syringe. The sample is then sent to the laboratory for testing.

You will usually be asked to rest for a short while after the test to allow everything to 'settle down' and then you will be able to go home. Most women say afterwards that the test was not painful, and that the thought of it was worse than the actual test. Some women say it feels more painful than any injection or blood test.

Although this test tells doctors the sex of the baby, doctors in some areas are very reluctant to give parents this information. This is because they are afraid that some parents might try to obtain an abortion if they were not happy with the sex of the baby. If this is indeed happening, there should be an investigation into who is carrying out abortions for such reasons. Restricting the information because some parents might seek an abortion is an example of tackling the problem from the wrong direction. If you find that the doctor is not willing to tell you the baby's sex you can approach the laboratory and, in writing, ask them to tell you. You should also complain to your Community Health Council (Scotland: Local Health Council; Northern Ireland: District Committee) and ask them to raise the matter on your behalf.

In the majority of areas women will have had two AFP blood tests before they are offered amniocentesis. If the first blood test showed high AFP levels the test should be repeated. If the levels in the second test are still high then you can decide whether or not you want to go ahead and have an amniocentesis. A high AFP does not necessarily mean that your baby has a chromosome disorder, women expecting twins or whose baby is older than is estimated also produce high levels of AFP.

The amniocentesis test for Down's syndrome is very accurate, 90 per cent; the spina bifida test has an accuracy around 80 to 90 per cent.

Over 25,000 women a year have this particular test. It is estimated that one woman in every 100–200 may miscarry because of the test (over and above those women who would have miscarried anyway). It is not known why this happens and there is no way of predicting which women are likely to miscarry because of the test.

There is also evidence suggesting that the test increases the risk of babies having difficulties with breathing after delivery. Fortunately this risk is rare and treatable, although it is not known what the long-term consequences may be.

The chance of having a Down's syndrome baby are:

Mother's age	The chances
25	1 in 1,500
30	1 in 800
35	1 in 350
36	1 in 300
37	1 in 200
38	1 in 170

39	1 in 140
40	1 in 100
45	1 in 30

AIDS - ACQUIRED IMMUNE DEFICIENCY SYNDROME

This is a disease which can develop as a result of an HIV-viral infection (human immunodeficiency virus). Not everyone who catches the virus goes on to develop AIDS, some people do not have any symptoms but carry the virus.

Some Health Authorities have introduced anonymous AIDS testing in a few trial areas. A small sample of the mother's blood is sent, in an unmarked container, for separate testing. The Authorities hope that they will eventually obtain data about the spread of AIDS amongst the general population. One assumes that they will use this information to determine what action they can take to educate and protect the population against this very serious disease.

Some Health Authorities are screening mothers' blood for AIDS antibodies, without first seeking their permission, and it is not being done anonymously. Such screening may, on the face of it, appear to be 'a good thing' but without giving women very careful counselling about the implications of having this screening, such action is highly questionable and leaves the Health Authorities at risk of having legal action for assault. It appears that the proposal to test every pregnant woman is being backed, primarily, to stop the spread of the disease by identifying those who have antibodies, but there is no evidence that such a course of action would be successful. There is a period when a woman may be infected but has not yet developed the HIV (human immunodeficiency virus) antibodies and in such cases the disease will not be detected. There are people with antibodies who have lived for years without developing AIDS, although some people may develop less severe illnesses which are not fatal. There is no cure to date and as long as that person is alive (even if they are well) they are infectious.

There is nothing whatsoever that can be done for a woman carrying the HIV antibodies apart from offering a termination of pregnancy, although there are no studies to show that termination makes any difference to the ultimate lifespan of the woman. What does seem to happen (according to American studies) is that in subsequent pregnancies the woman seems to have a higher incidence of developing symptoms of the disease. No one knows why, but it has been suggested that each pregnancy offers a further threat to the immune system.

It is claimed that were a mother found to be HIV-positive the information would be kept strictly confidential. There have been, however, many examples of breaches of confidentiality in the past; with such an emotive issues as AIDS it is doubtful that confidentiality would be maintained for long.

For the mother the implications of being HIV-positive are horrendous. Quite apart from the shock of being diagnosed as a carrier of a disease for which there is no cure, she will not be able to obtain life insurance nor would she be able to get a mortgage.

Screening all women for antibodies is not the answer. A great deal more attention needs to be given to the standards of hygiene in hospitals, bearing in mind the fact that large numbers of women already leave hospital with hospital-borne infections. Hospitals are, in general, far grubbier than most people's homes and there clearly needs to be a general tightening-up of standards of hygiene. There have been proposals that for all births midwives should wear goggles, overgowns, boots and require the partner to 'gown up' as well. Such proposals are an over-reaction. Of course it is necessary for health care workers to take great care that they do not get contaminated with blood or body fluids (including amniotic fluid). It would be sensible, therefore, for midwives and doctors to wear some eye protection, to be careful about any cuts or abrasions they may have and perhaps to stop handling maternity pads.

Some babies born to mothers who have developed HIV or AIDS have also caught the disease. A pregnant woman can pass the virus on to her baby in the womb and through breast milk (in about 25 to 30 per cent of cases). It is also possible that the route of infection is a foetal scalp electrode. Yet there have been no recommendations to stop using foetal scalp electrodes on babies in areas where there are many high-risk women.

City and Hackney Health Authority have introduced routine testing at the antenatal clinics. Although it is supposed to be 'voluntary' pregnant women are being strongly 'encouraged' (medico-speak for pressured) to agree to have the test. If they do not the midwives and doctors treat them as though they are HIV-positive. Particular pressure is being put on women wanting a home birth since they are told that the midwives may feel ambivalent about delivering a woman who has not been tested.

As with some other antenatal tests there is a high false positive rate. A study in Norway showed that out of 120,000 women tested, nine were found to be HIV-positive, five of these were already known to be positive. The worrying aspect of this was that 120 women were told they were HIV-positive after the test. With a second, more sensitive test, they were found in fact to be negative. The anxiety this raised for the women and their families was very high, most of the women continued to believe the result of the first test and believed they were carrying an 'infected' baby. In addition to the false positive rate appearing to be alarmingly high, there is also the high level of anxiety caused by having the test, even if the result is negative.

Midwives and doctors need to decide how they are going to deal with *all* pregnant women and babies in the light of what they know about AIDS. The main point, however, is that if a high standard of care is offered for all women, the staff will be protected, too, and will run very little risk. A great deal more thought needs to go into such action, preferably without the hysteria that has accompanied some proposals.

If, however, you have been told that you are HIV-positive, and are worried about breach of confidentiality, you can ask for a home birth. If midwives and doctors are truly worried about possible cross-infection they will recognise that giving birth at home will greatly limit this risk, and will also ensure a greater level of confidentiality for the woman.

You have every right to refuse to have your blood taken for AIDS testing (anonymously or not). If you are within the risk groups for AIDS and are worried about it there are a number of organisations which will give free confidential advice and counselling. They are separate from the hospitals and doctors:

- National AIDS Helpline – a free telephone service for people seeking advice: Tel: 0800 567-123
- Action on AIDS Team, St Leonard's Hospital, Nuttall Street, London N1, Tel. 071-739 8484 ext 4659
- Worried Well, 1st Floor, Milton Court Centre, Moor Lane, London EC2Y 9BN Tel: 071-601 7357

BLOOD PRESSURE

Throughout your pregnancy and at every check-up you will have your blood pressure taken; the result will be recorded on your co-operation card, or in your case notes if you are fortunate enough to live in an area where the women are given their case notes. Your blood pressure will be taken with a machine called a sphygmomanometer (an almost unpronounceable name). The midwife will wrap a cuff around your forearm and pump up the cuff. This constricts the artery in your arm and the machine can then detect the pressure. The midwife will read a meter (a bit like a wall thermometer). The mercury starts at the top, and as she releases the pressure the mercury falls. Experienced midwives can often read the blood pressure reading at amazing speed and you (if she has put the meter in a position where you can see it) will probably have a great deal of difficulty in seeing what it is she is looking at! As the mercury falls, it hiccoughs at a point which will give her the upper blood pressure reading (the systolic pressure). It then falls a little further and gives a second hiccough (the diastolic pressure). If you could not see what the readings were you can ask the midwife to tell you.

In some areas, midwives have electronic sphygmomanometers. These still have the cuff, but instead of a meter, the midwife holds what looks like a small clock with a second hand. This machine makes reading blood pressures much easier.

Normal blood pressure (bp) is anywhere within a range of 95/60 to 135/85. In order to determine what is normal for you, the midwife will take your bp at each appointment during the antenatal period. She will be looking to see if your bp suddenly rises and if it remains high. For example, if your bp rose from 95/60 to 100/80 then she would want to take it again, a little later, so see if it was just a sudden rise or whether it remained high. If it remained high, she would then want to discuss with you what action ought to be taken.

A rise in the upper bp reading is not as important as a rise in the lower figure, because the upper figure is affected by stressful circumstances and is often of a temporary nature.

Many women find that each time they go to the antenatal clinic their blood pressure goes up. This can often be due to stress and anxiety of attending the clinic. If you have rushed into the antenatal clinic late for your appointment, clutching a fractious toddler and worried about how you are going to get back in time to collect your eldest child from school, you are very likely to send your blood pressure through the roof! Apart from asking for the test to be done again, you might also wish to consider having your antenatal care in a less stressful environment. If this is the case, you can ask for a reading to be taken in your own home, or you can ask for the reading to be taken again in twenty minutes, after you have had a sit-down and a rest.

BLOOD TESTS

A blood sample is usually taken at the first antenatal visit in order to determine your blood type, to establish whether or not you have Rhesus blood type, to check whether you have rubella (German measles) antibodies and whether you have syphilis, gonorrhea or some of the more common sexually transmitted diseases. Fortunately, all these tests can be done on one sample of blood!

AFP blood test

Some women may be offered a further blood test called an serum alpha-fetoprotein test. This is done between 16 and 18 weeks. A high level of AFP may suggest that the baby has a congential handicap (e.g. spina bifida). This test, however, is not very accurate. Of those women with raised AFPs, who have an amniocentesis only 10 per cent will actually have handicapped babies. A high AFP result may be due to a number of factors, such as twins or an error over dates, so if you have a high AFP you should ask for a second test. If that test shows high levels of AFP you should then consider whether or not you wish to have an amniocentesis.

CHORIONIC VILLUS SAMPLING

Chorionic villus sampling (CVS) is the latest technique developed to detect some genetic diseases. The procedure is carried out between the ninth and eleventh week of gestation and should the procedure confirm a genetic defect, the mother will be offered an early abortion.

The test is carried out as an outpatient test; you do not have to be admitted to hospital. An ultrasound scan will be done to show the position of the developing pregnancy. You will need a full bladder for the scan.

Your vagina will be cleaned with an antiseptic solution and a thin tube is passed through the cervix (neck of the womb) guided to the right place by the ultrasound scan (this will feel rather like having an internal examination). A tiny fragment from the chorionic tissue is gently sucked into the tube and removed, then sent to the laboratory for testing. The chorionic tissue is what surrounds the embryo at this stage in pregnancy, and some of it will later form the placenta. Only a very small bit is removed, about the size of a few grains of rice. Some hospital employ a different method of taking these samples, using a needle through the abdomen, similar to the way amniocentesis is done. Both methods seem to work well.

The advantage of the technique is that if a damaged foetus is detected, an abortion can be offered and carried out earlier than an abortion following amniocentesis. Clearly an early abortion is a simpler procedure than one carried out later in pregnancy. The disadvatage is that, to date, CVS has a slightly higher miscarriage rate than amniocentesis and its diagnostic accuracy is less good than amniocentesis.

ELECTRONIC FOETAL HEART MONITORING IN PREGNANCY

Sometimes electronic foetal monitoring is used in pregnancy. The most common form of monitoring the baby's heartbeat is for the midwife to listen with a Pinard stethescope (it looks like a small ear trumphet – often wooden or plastic, sometimes metal). Experienced midwives are very good at this type of monitoring but their skills are being lost as a result of the routine use of electronic foetal monitoring or monitoring by ultrasound with a Sonicaid (a small, hand-held monitor, sometimes called a Doptone).

There is no justification at all for using electronic foetal monitoring in pregnancy. Indeed, four properly controlled studies have shown that the mortality rates were *higher* when electronic foetal monitoring was used in late pregnancy. Despite the evidence many women are asked to agree to a twenty-minute period of monitoring during the pregnancy!

If you are asked to agree to a short period of electronic monitoring you could ask the staff for their reasons and then draw their attention to the research. You do not have to agree to this if you do not want to have it done.

An electronic foetal monitor which involves a buckle strapped across your abdomen or the hand-held version both use ultrasound; although the intensity of the ultrasound beam is less than that used when you have an ultrasound examination showing a 'picture' of your baby on a screen.

(See Chapter 11, 'Common obstetric procedures and technologies', p.107 for further information about electronic foetal monitoring.)

FOETAL MOVEMENT COUNTING

In many areas women are being asked if they would like to keep a record of the numbers of episodes of kicking they experience during their pregnancy. It is usually carried out during the thirtieth to fourtieth weeks, over a period of twelve hours, or until ten kicking episodes have occurred, or, in some areas, the women are asked to count for a period of one hour.

It has been known for a century that reduced movements can indicate that the baby is not doing well. A scheme was developed in which the mother counted the numbers of kicking episodes but it was found that there were false alarms because it did not take account in the variations in activity between foetuses. Everyone knows that some babies are very much more active than others.

Some women are delighted to keep a 'kick chart', others find them very threatening and worry a great deal more. Research has shown that less than one in a thousand women might benefit from foetal movement counting in terms of the prevention of late foetal death. You have the right to refuse to keep a 'kick chart' if you do not want to do so.

ULTRASOUND

Some 100 million people throughout the world are walking around having had scans before they were born, and there has

never been a shred of evidence that it does harm. (Professor Stuart Campbell as quoted in *The Sunday Times*, 10 June 1984).
The data on clinical efficacy and safety do not allow a recommendation for routine screening at this time, there is a need for multi-disciplinary randomised controlled clinical trials for an adequate assessment. (World Health Organisation, 1984).

Women are currently exposed to ultrasound scanning periodically throughout their pregnancies, sometimes as early as six to eight weeks' gestation, and are frequently told that ultrasound is absolutely safe. Books on childbirth frequently reinforce that opinion, for example, *A New Life* by Dr David Harvey states 'Ultrasound is a completely safe technique which provides detailed information of the earliest changes in uterine growth and the development of the foetus.' This statement may well prove to be true, but the medical profession has not conducted any long-term studies to find out if it is safe. Until those studies have been done it is sensible to use ultrasound only when necessary and not subject the whole population to its use. If there are long-term effects of ultrasound then the minimum number of women and babies will have been put at risk.

It is hardly surprising, therefore, if many women feel that they are not being properly cared for if they have not had an ultrasound scan. The majority of British women are totally unaware that there are anxieties about ultrasound, and that statements about its absolute safety cannot be supported by carefully evaluated scientific evidence.

Ultrasound was first developed to detect flaws in the hulls of ships. Its development in obstetric care followed a visit to a Glasgow shipyard by an obstetrician who realised that if it could find cracks in ships' hulls then it could be used in pregnancy to 'see' into the woman's abdomen. Since its introduction some thirty years ago it has been widely and enthusiastically taken up by the medical profession and has been adapted for a wide variety of uses.

Ultrasound can be used to detect twins, ectopic pregnancies (where the egg grows in the fallopian tube), assess many foetal abnormalities, foetal growth retardation, foetal breathing movements, heart function and guide other procedures such as chorionic villus sampling and amniocentesis. Its accuracy in detecting these conditions, however, depends a great deal on the skill of the operator. Its major use is to establish a woman's dates and check the foetal heart beat with a Doptone or Sonicaid during pregnancy.

In 1979 the Association for Improvements in the Maternity Services (AIMS) became aware of American studies which suggested that ultrasound was not the benign procedure the obstetricians claimed it was and it began to question its routine use in maternity care.

Ultrasound is a classic example of an unevaluated technique which has been introduced into maternity care in an uncontrolled fashion, and little or no effort being made to check the possible effects of ultrasound over the long term.

From the limited amount of scientific evidence available it is almost certain that ultrasound does not cause any gross abnormality or problem; these would have been detected by now with the numbers of women and babies who have been exposed to ultrasound. The problem, however, is that no-one has any idea about the possible long-term subtle effects that ultrasound might have on babies.

A study in America (Stark *et al*, 1984) has suggested that there is a connection between ultrasound exposure in utero (in the womb) and dyslexia (difficulties with reading, spelling and communication). Although not a well-designed study, it is one of the few to look at future problems with ultrasound, and it sounds a warning bell we would be unwise to ignore.

The majority of medical commentators, however, are not so cautious; they have continued to assert the safety of ultrasound and have produced reports that are misleading and staggering in their hypocrisy. On the one hand claims are made that ultrasound reduces perinatal mortality and handicap, on the other the Royal College of Obstetricians and Gynaecologists' (RCOG) own report states

> There is a serious lack of prospective studies to provide evidence that routine ultrasound scanning as opposed to selective scanning on clinical indication reduces perinatal mortality and handicap or reduces maternal morbidity.

The RCOG Report goes on to state that

> we find no study in the entire body of biomedical ultrasound which clearly demonstrates that there is any effect on the mammalian foetus from pulsed echo ultrasound of diagnostic intensities.

AIMS took issue with the RCOG report and published a critique which commented:

> As the studies have not been done then they are hardly likely to find evidence. It is rather like looking for an elephant at the

bottom of the Indian Ocean; having failed to find one it is then confidently stated that elephants do not exist.

The RCOG Report also states that:

Studies on rats demonstrate that ultrasound can cause foetal abnormalities and growth retardation depending on the stage of development and insonations, . . . expert opinion attributes these effects to ultrasound heating which does not occur with diagnostic ultrasound. (Note: When ultrasound is used in experiments it is used at high intensities and when used at that level heat is produced.)

It is of considerable concern that the RCOG is not prepared to accept that indications of anomalies in animals should be taken as an indication of possible risk to people. There is a parallel with the testing of new drugs:

After animal tests have been accepted the next major hurdle is the clinical trial. There is no substitute for using the drug on man, for no matter how rigorous the animal test procedures, some effects will slip through. Practolol passed all the required animal tests; and with thalidomide it was found that the polyneuritis it induced is unique to man, and *some effort was necessary to reproduce its foetus-deforming effect in laboratory animals*' (our emphasis) (extract from *Cured to Death* by Arabella Melville and Colin Johnson).

The RCOG claims that any effects found in animals are produced by using ultrasound at a far higher level than is used in clinical practice. Unfortunately, the equipment manufacturers are unable to monitor the output levels of their machines. It is known that ultrasound machines 'peak', so how does the RCOG know that the equipment does not exceed the range of diagnostic levels?

Furthermore, in their enthusiasm to increase the uses of diagnostic ultrasound, obstetricians are now developing techniques which use two and three ultrasound beams at the same time. How much ultrasound are the mother and baby being exposed to when they are subjected to extensive periods of ultrasound examination by this method?

Another new development is a scanner which allows obstetricians to conduct vaginal scanning as early as six weeks into the pregnancy. It involves using a probe ten to fifteen centimetres in length which they introduce into the vagina to around two or three centimetres from the cervix. It uses a higher frequency of ultrasound waves which the obstetricians claim produce an 'exceptionally clear picture'. They also claim that although this form of scanning uses a vaginal probe it 'carries no risk of miscarriage' (*Mother and Baby*), May 1990). Once again, obstetricians are being economical with the truth. There is no scientific evidence which will support such a claim, and since the *Mother and Baby* article an American research paper has shown that, amongst a group of patients at risk for pre-term birth, the risk of early miscarriage was *doubled* when ultrasound was used (Lorenz, 1990). Those who are concerned about this unevaluated technology are particularly worried about its use during early pregnancy which is such a sensitive period in the development of the foetus.

Ultrasound, when properly used, is capable of detecting a wide range of abnormalities, this advantage, however, is not without problems. The RCOG report lists a range of abnormalities that were detected and went on to state that:

> Ultrasound was shown in the study to have a 100 per cent sensitivity in diagnosing craniospinal defects but unfortunately one normal foetus was terminated following a false positive diagnosis of hydrocephaly.

The report does not state whether or not all the babies with the conditions listed were aborted, although one assumes that they were. If they were aborted how many of them would have died anyway during the pregnancy or at birth? What was the effect on the mothers of these abortions? Would that have been better or worse than leaving the baby alone? The healthy foetus who was aborted shows how even in a very advanced ultrasound screening pro-gramme errors occur. How great is the increase in errors in those departments where the staff are less trained and are using less up-to-date equipment?

The medical profession in this country continues to use ultra-sound as a routine on the vast majority of pregnant woman, with little evidence that ultrasound is effective when used in this way. It is certainly expensive, the Department of Health (DH) is currently spending anything upwards of £14 million a year on it. Many of the examinations are unnecessary and any women agreeing to expose her baby to ultrasound should insist that a record is kept of the exposure. (A standard record is listed at the end of this chapter.)

Without doubt, ultrasound is very valuable for specific problems during the pregnancy. Any women who suddenly starts bleeding will welcome the invention of ultrasound, but that is no justification for exposing all women and babies to it.

It seems absurd that when insufficient funds are available for many necessary procedures so much money is being spent on an unevaluated technology.

AIMS has campaigned for many years for the use of ultrasound to be restricted to those women who really need it. In October 1984 the Under Secretary of State for Health, John Patten, stated in a letter to AIMS that 'given the publicity there has been recently about the possible risks of ultrasound scanning we (i.e. the Department of Health) would not expect any Health Authority to be advocating screening during pregnancy for all mothers as a routine procedure'.

The World Health Organisation has also issued a policy statement on ultrasound exposure:

The WHO stresses the health technologies should be thoroughly evaluated prior to their widespread use. Ultrasound screening during pregnancy is now in widespread use without sufficient evaluation. Research has demonstrated its efficacy for certain complications of pregnancy but the published material does not justify the routine use of ultrasound in pregnancy care.

There is also insufficient information with regard to the safety of ultrasound use during pregnancy. There is, as yet, no comprehensive multi-disciplinary assessment of ultrasound use during pregnancy including: clinical efficacy, psycho-social effects, ethical consideration, legal implications, cost benefit, and safety. This lack of information makes decision making and priority setting with regard to ultrasound use during pregnancy difficult.

A relevant document which provides guidance and policy in this matter is the US Concensus statement *Diagnostic Ultrasound Imaging in Pregnancy* published by the National Institute of Health in 1984. The WHO organisation can, in principle, support this statement including their views that: the data on clinical efficacy and safety do not allow a recommendation for routine screening at this time; there is a need for multidisciplinary randomised controlled clinical trials for an adequate assessment.

The WHO strongly endorses the principle of informed choice with regard to technology use. The health-care providers have the moral responsibility to fully inform each woman prior to an ultrasound examination as to the clinical indication for ultrasound, its hoped for benefit, its potential risks and alternative available if any.

Many members of the medical profession in this country have ignored this suggestion. Such is the complacency about ultrasound that no records are kept of those who have been exposed. Had this been done from the very beginning it would now be possible to answer some of the questions about ultrasound safety.

Many parents who have anxieties about routine ultrasound exposure are heavily pressured into consenting to its use, often they are made to feel they are being negligent in refusing the treatment, sometimes they are told that if they refuse and the baby is born with a serious complication (a very rare occurrence) they will be responsible.

Your rights

You have every right to refuse to expose your baby to an ultrasound examination. If you feel that the examination is being suggested merely as a routine, you should ask the staff to justify their reasons for recommending it. The final decision, however, is yours. To those who suggest that should the baby be born with an abnormality that could have been detected by ultrasound it will be entirely your fault, you could point out that their punitive attitude does not seem to apply to those members of the medical profession who have aborted fit and healthy babies wrongly diagnosed by ultrasound examination, and as no statistical data is available to identify the risks of that happening, the profession is in no position to criticise your decision.

Many women who want to have an ultrasound examination and wish to bring their partners, or a friend, with them are often told that this is impossible. A father or friend has no legal right to be present and the only leverage the mother has is to refuse to have the ultrasound done unless her partner is there. This is a difficult position to adopt when one wants the examination, but those women who have put their feet down have usually found that the staff have relented. Some hospitals, like St Mary's Portsmouth, will allow a partner in but will not allow any other relative or friend to come. This particularly discriminates against the single woman or the woman whose husband or partner is not able to attend. Other hospitals will allow the husband or partner in for the first ultrasound examination, but refuse to have them in for the second. You can deal with this by using similar tactics, in both instances you could also write to the the CHC (Scotland: Local health council; N. Ireland: District Committee), and the Chair of the District Health Authority (in Scotland, Health District; in Northern Ireland, Health and Social District), your MP, and complain about the hospital staff's attitude.

If you decide to have an ultrasound examination, foetal monitoring or consent to the use of a hand-held Doptone or Sonicaid, you may wish to impress upon those carrying out the examinations the importance of keeping adequate records of their practice. You have the right, therefore, to insist that they complete a record of ultrasound exposure (see p. 32) and attach it to your case notes. In this way we shall begin to develop records of exposures in the UK and when the medical profession finally gets around to assessing the effects of ultrasound it will have some evidence available. You can obtain A4 size copies of this form and other information about ultrasound from the Association for Improvements in the Maternity Services, Goose Green Barn, Much Hoole, Preston, Lancashire, PR4 4TD, or you can take this book along to a photocopying shop.

RECORD OF ULTRASOUND EXPOSURE

Doctor or midwife

The following procedure requiring the use of ultrasound

....

is necessary to obtain the following information

....

which is needed for the further management of this pregnancy. The indication for the procedure is

....

To my knowledge there is no current alternative method available to obtain this information that carries less risk to (mother's name)

.... and/or her fetus(es).

Signature (Doctor's or midwife's) ....
Name (in Capitals) ....

Details of ultrasound exposure

....

Manufacturer and model of ultrasound equipment

....

Type of ultrasound ....

Intensity of exposure (W/cm2 or mW/cm2)* ....

Length of exposure ....

Time commenced ....Time completed ....

Name of hospital ....or clinic of ....

Procedure carried out by (name in capitals) ....

Signature ....Date ....

Position ....

*Watts per square centimetre exposed

URINE TESTS

During your pregnancy you will have your urine tested regularly in order to check for the presence of sugar in the urine, a possible indication of gestational diabetes, and the presence of albumen (protein) which is one symptom of pre-eclampsia. If you have a urine infection, the urine will be sent to a laboratory for testing and the infection can then be treated.

Later in your pregnancy you may be asked to do an oestriol test. This involves collecting urine over a 24-hour period. Oestriol tests are not particularly reliable, and, on the basis of available studies, there is no evidence to suggest any benefit from carrying out oestriol tests. Research has shown that the tests 'were not sensitive enough to detect the majority of pregnancies destined to have an adverse outcome, and that a great many women with normal pregnancies falsely appeared to be at risk'.

If it is suggested that you have an oestriol test you can ask them to indicate what scientific evidence they have to support such a suggestion, and why do they wish to do it in your case. You have the right to refuse to have it done.

X-RAYS

There was a time when obstetricians were recommending that all women should have X-rays during their pregnancies, however, the profession is now more cautious about using X-rays on pregnant women.

Wherever possible X-rays should be avoided in pregnancy, but women who are believed to be suffering from cephalic disproportion are often advised to have an X-ray. *Effective Care in Pregnancy and Childbirth* states

Neither X-ray nor clinical pelvimetry have been shown to predict cephalopelvic disproportion with sufficient accuracy to justify elective caesarean section for cephalic presentations. Cephalopelvic disproportion is best diagnosed by a carefully monitored trial of labour, and X-ray pelvimetry should seldom, if ever, be necessary.

Computed tomographic pelvimetry, which greatly reduces the radiation exposure to the foetus, has been found in two small studies to be easier to perform, and in the measurement of a model pelvis, probably more accurate than conventional X-ray pelvimetry.

If it is suggested that you need a pelvic X-ray during your pregnancy you can ask for a second opinion, or refuse. If you find that you have to have a dental X-ray you can ask the dentist for a lead apron to protect your baby and your ovaries. Research shows that a significant number of children with leukaemia and some other cancers were exposed to X-rays in utero.

4
CHOOSING YOUR CHILDBIRTH PROFESSIONAL

CONSULTANT OBSTETRICIANS

Consultant obstetricians are experts in abnormality, they have little experience of normal childbirth and their training specifically focuses on the abnormal. This results in many of them having a lack of understanding or knowledge of normal labour and childbirth and a general lack of sympathy for those women who believe that for the majority childbirth is a normal physiological event.

Women who book a hospital birth with a consultant obstetrician are rarely told that they have a choice. The GP usually automatically refers you to his/her favourite consultant. You can however suggest that s/he refers you to the consultant you want to see. If s/he refuses to do so you can change GP or simply refuse to agree to his/her choice. Once a GP has taken you on for maternity care s/he has the responsibility of booking you into a suitable hospital, so s/he will be under some pressure to find you someone you want. The pressure will increase as time goes by if you still have not agreed to a specific booking.

Before you agree to be booked with a specific consultant you should find out what his/her policies are, by speaking to other mothers who have had babies in that hospital, by writing to the local Community Health Council and writing to the Hospital Administrator and asking him/her.

Consultant obstetricians head a team, and s/he sets the policy for her/his staff. Find out what the other obstetricians' policies are, and how they differ from each other. You will then be in a better position to judge which one will give you the kind of care you would prefer.

The majority of women rarely see their consultant obstetrician, they are either busy with the 'problem' cases or very involved with their private practice. Occasionally, women are cared for by obstetricians who are arrogant, self-opinionated and downright rude. You do not have to tolerate this.

One woman refused to have an induction of labour, so the consultant hurled the case notes down on her bed and informed her that if she was not prepared to take his advice he was not prepared to attend her. He then turned on his heel and marched out of the ward closely followed by his entourage of medical students and midwives. The woman was scared stiff and immediately agreed to the induction. Unfortunately, she did not know that she could have asked to see the Supervisor of Midwives, whom she could then inform that she was withdrawing from consultant care and required the midwives to look after her instead. (It is perfectly possible to have midwifery care only.) If a situation arose where the women required the attention of a consultant the midwives would call one (and he would have to attend).

Had a similar incident happened during pregnancy the woman could ask her GP to refer her to another obstetrician or to midwifery care only. She should also inform the consultant that she is no longer prepared to be attended by him/her and send a copy of her letter to the hospital administrator. If the GP refuses to refer her to another obstetrician she can either change GPs or write to the hospital administrator herself, with a copy to the Regional Health Authority. The Regional Health Authority holds consultants' contracts and it is important for them to understand the quality of obstetrician they are employing.

GENERAL PRACTITIONERS

General practitioners are local community doctors who are responsible for providing 24-hour medical cover. It is important for you to establish your GP's qualifications if you want him/her to look after you during your pregnancy, labour and delivery. Any GP can look after you, but it is preferable to be cared for by a GP who has additional obstetric training and is, therefore, on the Obstetrics List. Check with the list which is held in most main post offices, or telephone the Family Health Services Authority (FHSA) (Scotland: the Primary Care Division of the Health Board; Northern Ireland: Central Services Agency). Whether or not your present GP has the additional qualifications you have the right to change to a GP who is on the obstetric list for your maternity care only.

Some of the GPs on the Obstetric List are very enthusiastic about childbirth and are not only actively involved in delivering babies in their local GP unit but are also involved with home births.

If you are choosing a home birth you do not need to approach a GP, you can book directly with the midwives. If however you have a GP who is known to be enthusiastic about home births s/he is to be encouraged and supported (they are very rare beings). If you particularly want GP care for a home birth you could contact the Association of General Practice Maternity Care. They have a list of GPs who are interested in home births and could tell you whether or not you have one in your area.

The quality of GPs offering shared care varies considerably. Unfortunately few Health Authorities have defined precisely what care the GP should give under this system and occasionally women receive a very poor standard of care indeed. If you feel that the quality of care you are receiving from your GP is poor you should contact your FHSA (Scotland: Primary Care Division of the Health Board, Northern Ireland: Central Services Agency) and inform them. You can then also transfer to another GP or book for midwifery care only. The FHSA will tell you how to transfer and if you want to change to midwifery care you can do this by writing to the Supervisor of Midwives at your local hospital.

HEALTH VISITORS

Health visitors are nurses who may have, but do not need to have, midwifery qualifications, and who have undertaken a special course in health visiting which includes child care and development. The midwife is responsible for your care up to twenty-eight days postnatally, after that the health visitor will be available (although in many cases care is transferred earlier at around ten days, and longer if you or your baby are not well). She will be concerned about your and your baby's physical and emotional well-being. She will visit you at home at a mutually convenient time and is available to give you help and advice. She will have details of the local clinics, mother and baby groups and will be able to advise you about developmental checks for the baby as well as details of immunisation and vaccinations. Health visitors can be particularly helpful if you have any specific problems postnatally which you want to discuss. You are, however, under no obligation to see her if you do not want to. Nor are you under any obligation to attend the local clinics or mother and baby groups.

MIDWIVES

A midwife is a person who . . . must be able to give the necessary supervision, care and advice to women during pregnancy, labour and the postpartum period, to conduct deliveries on her own responsibility and to care for the newborn and the infant. This care includes preventative measures, the detection of abnormal conditions in mother and child, the procurement of medical assistance and the execution of emergency measures in the absence of medical help. She has an important task in health counselling and education, not only for the patients, but also within the family and the community . . . (from the definition of a midwife adopted by the International Confederation of Midwives and International Federation of Gynaecologists and Obstetricians).

What the above says essentially is that midwives are the experts in normality. There are problems, however, with the way in which midwives have been trained and midwifery is organised in many parts of the country. Unfortunately, there are two types of midwives, obstetric nurses and midwives. Both are called midwives, but obstetric nurses are those who generally work in hospitals, do not give continuity of care and have one specific area of work. She might be employed in the antenatal clinic as an escort, urine tester and doctor's chaperone, or she might be on the labour ward carrying out the obstetrician's policies, or on the postnatal ward. Only a few hospitals have midwifery teams where the midwife has her own case load and is responsible for the care of her clients throughout the antenatal, birth and postnatal periods.

Over the last ten years or so there have been considerable tensions between these two groups, those midwives who want to use their skills to the full, and those who are quite happy acting as a handmaiden and being told what to do. The latter are often very threatened by any suggestion that they should revert to their full role of providing total care for low-risk women.

This split within the profession causes considerable problems for women who are seeking the best care for themselves and their babies.

Increasingly, however, many midwives have been very active in stimulating their colleagues into questioning the way in which they are (mis)used in many Health Authorities, and have been encouraging them to reclaim their true role as experts in normality.

Those midwives who are members of the Association of Radical Midwives are generally midwives who believe that childbirth is essentially a normal physiological event. They believe that their role is to help and support the mother to encourage the progress of birth without unnecessary interference.

There have been a number of studies which show that continuity of care provided by midwives results in greater satisfaction from the mothers, less technological interventions and fitter babies, and no adverse effects on foetal outcomes.

If you are planning to give birth in hospital, and you want to give birth with a midwife you know, you can book a 'domino delivery' (see page 57). Otherwise you will be attended by whichever midwife is on duty, and you may never have met her before.

If you are planning a home birth booking a midwife of your choice is much simpler (see pages 43-5), although in many cases you may find that there is only a one in ten chance of having someone you know.

The majority of midwives are kind, considerate and charming people who are doing their best to give you the very best of care, sometimes in difficult circumstances. Many hospitals are grossly understaffed and many midwives are working under considerable pressure.

Sometimes women find themselves being attended by someone they dislike or who has little sympathy with the childbirth methods they want to use. In these circumstances the woman has every right to dismiss her attendant.

If you have booked a home birth you have plenty of opportunity to get to know your midwife, and if you find that she is not very helpful or you do not get on you have plenty of opportunity to take action before labour begins. If you have booked a hospital delivery you may not meet the midwife before you are in labour, or they may change shifts in the middle. Obviously, taking action in these circumstances is difficult but that does not prevent you from doing anything at all. You could point out to her that you are not happy with her care and suggest that she alters her attitude. If she does not you can refuse to be attended by her. A midwife cannot abandon a women in the middle of her labour, she has a legal duty to attend and she will, therefore have to contact the senior midwife on duty, or the Supervisor of Midwives, and ask for a replacement. If she refuses to do this you can insist on calling the Supervisor of Midwives yourself (or your partner can do it for you).

Male midwives

All midwifery training schools have now to accept male midwives if they apply for training. The staff should make it clear to you, before you go into hospital, that you might be attended by a male midwife and that you may decide whether or not you wish to be attended by them.

You have an absolute right to refuse to be attended by a male midwife (or a male doctor for that matter) if you wish. You can make it clear before you go into hospital by adding your consent or refusal to your letter to the hospital.

PAEDIATRICIANS

Paediatricians are doctors who specialise in the care of babies and children. Once a baby is delivered the obstetrician's job has finished and the paediatrician's job begins. Many women do not see the paediatrician, far too many hospitals remove the baby after delivery for a paediatric check. You can insist that the check is carried out in your presence and the paediatrician asked to come to you.

It is a common good practice for a paediatrician to be present for the birth of any baby whose condition before birth is giving cause for concern, or where the birth is assisted, for example forceps or ventouse, particularly if the reason for these interventions is that the baby is distressed.

Good paediatricians will always introduce themselves to the mother and, if time permits, explain their role.

5

CHOOSING A HOME BIRTH

The practice of delivering nearly all babies in hospital has contributed to the dramatic reduction in stillbirths and neonatal deaths and to the avoidance of many child handicaps (*Second Report of the Maternity Services Advisory Committee*, 1984).
There is no evidence to support the claim that the safest policy is for all women to give birth in hospital (Rona Campbell and Alison Macfarlane, 1989).

A great deal of misinformation has been given about home birth over the years. At one time all babies were born at home, but with the growth of hospitals and the greater influence of the medical profession over childbirth more and more women were persuaded to have their babies in hospital. The majority of government reports about childbirth recommended birth in hospital because it was 'safer'. None of them produced any evidence to substantiate that claim.

The real push to bring women into hospital came in the 1950s when there was a shortage of hospital beds and women who really *ought* to have had a hospital birth were not able to arrange a booking. Examination of the early journals of the Association for Improvements in the Maternity Services shows that it was anxious about the numbers of women who were giving birth in hospital corridors!

Having brought in the few women who needed to be in hospital, there was a drive to get *everyone* in, on the time-honoured principle that if x is a good thing for some then it must also be a good thing for all. Furthermore, getting more women into hospital ensured

more jobs for obstetricians and more women and babies on whom
they could practise medical procedures.

The hospitalisation of childbirth would have been 100 per cent
successful but for one woman – Margaret Whyte. She set up the
Society to Support Home Confinement, an organisation which gives
help, advice and support to those women who want a home birth.
Without her activities in the 1970s home birth would have been as
dead as the Dodo. When the childbirth groups finally woke up to
the fact that home birth was *almost* completely phased out, they
found that Margaret had been fighting a rearguard action for years.
Since then the childbirth groups have continually challenged the
profession to prove that hospital birth is safer than home birth and
substantiate their claims with scientific evidence. The profession
has not been able to do so. AIMS challenged the profession to
conduct a randomised controlled trial of home and hospital birth,
but the challenge was never taken up. There is a belief within the
profession that insufficient numbers of women would agree to take
part in such a study. This belief is erroneous: there are many
women who would be interested in taking part in a trial, if only as a
means of getting the home birth which is often vigorously opposed
by health authorities.

Because of the continual questioning of the validity of the
obstetricians' claims, that home birth is dangerous and hospital
birth is safe, a number of researchers started to examine these
questions.

The most important is Marjorie Tew, a statistician from Notting-
ham. She examined the statistical data from the 1958 and 1970
British Births Surveys and made adjustments for the proportions of
births in different risk categories (obstetricians often claim that
they have higher mortality rates because they have to deal with
more high-risk women). Her conclusion was that had women
stayed at home to have their babies at the same rates as they did in
the 1950s, the infant mortality rate today would be four points
lower than it is. This means that every year over 2,400 babies die
as *a direct result* of entering consultant units or teaching hospitals
to give birth. Marjorie argues that the infant mortality rate was
already falling when the obstetricians took over birth and what they
did was to *slow down* the fall in infant mortality rates. It would
have fallen even faster had they not hospitalised the majority of
women.

In 1984 Rona Campbell and her colleagues published a survey of
all the home births in England and Wales which took place in 1979.
They found that among the booked home births, the perinatal
mortality rate (stillbirths and babies that die up to six days after the
birth) was 4.1 per 1,000, compared with 67.8 per 1,000 for those

who booked consultant hospital deliveries and 196.6 per 1,000 for those who made no plans (the national mortality rate for all births was 14.6 per 1,000).

In 1988 the Ministry of Health introduced a new data collection system, but because of the failure of many health authorities to make proper returns it has not been possible to undertake a full analysis and update the 1979 data.

The latest review of the safety of home and hospital birth, *Where to be Born? The Debate and the Evidence*, has been published by the National Perinatal Epidemiology Unit, Oxford. In it Rona Campbell and Alison Macfarlane concluded that

> The available evidence does not support claims that, for the baby, the iatrogenic (doctor-caused) risks of obstetric inter- vention outweigh the possible benefits. At the same time, there is no evidence to support the claim that the shift to hospital delivery is responsible for the decline in perinatal mortality in England and Wales nor the claim that the safest policy is for all women to be delivered in hospital.

HOW TO ARRANGE A HOME BIRTH

> In many areas women seeking home birth will need the patience of Job, the courage of Joan of Arc and the political skill of a Metternich' (Jean Donnison, 1988).

It is the right of every woman to have a home birth, if she so wishes. The decision is hers, and hers alone. It does not depend upon the approval of the GP, the consultant or the midwife, although, clearly, a woman would listen to any professional advice before making up her mind and deciding what is best for herself and her baby.

Current statistical data show that for low-risk healthy women a home birth is safer than a hospital birth. There are, however, some rare conditions which would exclude a home birth e.g. a placenta praevia (where the position of the placenta prevents a normal vagina delivery).

To obtain a home birth a woman can take the following steps:

• Write to the Supervisor of Midwives (at your local maternity unit) stating that you intend having a home birth and asking her to provide you with a midwife.

You can book a home birth directly with the midwives. You do not need to ask your GP, your obstetricians, or anyone else for permission and unless you are sure that your GP is an enthusiast

for home births, it is far better to book with the midwives directly.
Your letter to the Supervisor of Midwives could be along the
following lines:

Dear Madam
I expect a baby sometime in (state month) and intend to give
birth at home. I have not approached my GP for support and I
shall not attempt to find a GP who will take me on. If you feel
that GP support is needed then I expect you to make the
necessary arrangements for adequate medical cover. I do not
intend becoming involved in that issue.
   Accordingly, I should be obliged if you would make the
necessary arrangements for a midwife to undertake my pregnancy and delivery care in my own home.
   I accept full responsibility for my decision to give birth at
home and I know that you accept the responsibility of providing me with a competent midwife fully backed up by such
facilities as are necessary to make the confinement as safe as
possible.

Yours faithfully

Copies to:
District Medical Officer (Scotland: Chief Administrative Medical
Officer)
Chair, District Health Authority (Scotland: Health District;
Northern Ireland: Health and Social Services District)
Chair, Community Health Council (Scotland: Local Health
Council; Northern Ireland: District Committee).

• If your GP is interested in doing home births (very few of them
  are), and does a lot of home births, then you can approach
  him/her and ask him/her if s/he would be prepared to provide
  cover for the home birth which you are booking with the midwives. If s/he is prepared to provide cover then your letter to the
  midwives could be along the following lines:

Dear Madam
I expect a baby sometime in (state month) and intend to give
birth at home. My GP (give name and address) has stated that
s/he is willing to offer me medical care for the birth.
   I should be obliged if you would make the necessary
arrangements for a midwife to undertake my pregnancy and
delivery care in my own home.

I accept full responsibility for my decision to give birth at home and I know that you accept the responsibility of providing me with a competent midwife fully backed up by such facilities as are necessary to make my confinement as safe as possible.

Yours sincerely

Copies should go to the:
District Medical Officer (Scotland: Chief Administrative Officer)
Chair, District Health Authority (Scotland: Health District; Northern Ireland: Health and Social Services District)
Chair, Community Health Council (Scotland: Local Health Council; Northern Ireland, District Committee).

Women are often told that they should obtain GP cover for the midwife. This is not their responsibility and they should not become involved with such arrangements. Midwives are the experts in normality and as such are qualified and competent to deliver babies at home without GP cover. Indeed, there are many midwives who feel that the involvement of an anxious GP who is not qualified to deliver babies at home (they have no midwifery qualifications) is a distinct liability and often results in mothers being admitted to hospital, not because there is a real problem but because of the anxieties of the GPs (which sometimes affect the midwives too). Those GPs who are GP obstetricians have qualified in the management of abnormal childbirth; very few of them have studied normal births – to do that they would need to take a midwifery course.
Some GPs resent women who book a home birth, or sign on with another GP for their maternity care (and many do), and have been known to strike them – and sometimes the whole family – off their list. If, however, the woman has already signed on for maternity care with the GP then s/he cannot strike her off without her consent or before applying to the FHSA for permission to do so.
Should s/he remove you without permission then you should write, within thirteen weeks, to the FHSA (Scotland: write within six weeks to the Primary Care Division of the Health Board; Northern Ireland: Central Services Agency) stating that s/he has struck you off, without your, or the FHSA's, permission and your GP is, therefore, in breach of contract.
There is, however, another problem which should be recognised. Because of the very low numbers of births taking place at home not many midwives are experienced at home deliveries. At present the

midwifery training programme does not equip midwives adequately
to deal with home births, so there are many midwives who find the
idea of doing home birth terrifying: their hospital training has
accustomed them to see birth as a high-risk event. In Scotland, the
problem is particularly bad because the practice of Scottish midwives does not meet English standards. Should there be a sudden
increase in home births in Scotland, there are very few midwives
sufficiently practised and confident to deal with them.

If you find you have a midwife who has little or no experience of
home births (she ought to have done at least six home births) you
can insist she bring a colleague with her. In that way not only will
she have some professional support, but you will be ensuring that
another midwife is learning about home births. In the 1940s
student midwives were trained by sending them out to do home
deliveries for first-time mothers on their own. Such training
developed confident and skilled midwives; perhaps it is time that
the scheme was re-introduced.

RESPONSIBILITY FOR A HOME BIRTH

Many Health Authorities seek to intimidate women by suggesting
that the responsibility for a home birth rests entirely on their
shoulders, and should anything go wrong the woman is liable.
Basingstoke and North Hampshire Health Authority had taken this
form of intimidation one step further. Their consent form stated:

> I . . . have been fully informed of the complications that may
> arise in connection with my pregnancy and the delivery of the
> child which I am carrying. . . . I will not consent to being
> admitted to hospital.
>
> In these circumstances, I fully understand and accept that
> neither my General Practitioner nor the Basingstoke and North
> Hampshire Health Authority nor any member of its medical,
> nursing or midwifery staff, can accept responsibility for any
> damage or injury which may be caused to myself or to my
> estates or my dependents or to the child, arising in any way
> whatsoever out of, or connected with my refusal to consent to
> myself being admitted to Hospital.
>
> I accordingly absolve my General Practitioner, the Basing-
> stoke and North Hampshire Health Authority, and its medical,
> nursing and midwifery staff from any liability to myself and
> estates or to my dependants in respect thereof.

This consent form's primary purpose is intimidation. Having failed
to intimidate women into hospital by requiring them to sign

consent forms stating that they take total responsibility for a home birth, this Health Authority has taken a further step by suggesting that the parents absolve the birth attendants of all responsibility. This they cannot do. After pressure from a local mother and AIMS this form was withdrawn and the Health Authority issued 'advice' to midwives.

Any women presented with such a form should refuse to sign it. If you feel, however, that you will suffer further harassment if you do not you can sign the form and add the following:

> I have not been advised of the increased risks to myself, and my baby, of hospital birth which sometimes results in dead or injured babies and can cause serious postnatal complications for mother and baby. This form has been signed under duress.

It is important to remember that it is rare for a serious or life-threatening event to occur with a booked home birth, but should one occur the midwife could only be liable had she acted negligently; and signing the above form would not alter that. If she acted in a professional manner and the outcome was a disaster then neither she nor the mother can be held responsible.

RESPONSIBILITY FOR HIGH-RISK WOMEN WHO INSIST ON A HOME BIRTH

The decision whether or not to have a home birth rests entirely with the mother. If she decides that she is going to have a home birth, even though she is truly a high-risk case, the Health Authority still has an obligation to provide a midwife. The midwife concerned would have informed the mother that she truly is at high risk and precisely what the reasons are for this professional opinion. Having identified a high-risk mother or baby, the midwife is then expected to take reasonable precautions so that should a crisis occur she is in the best position to deal with it.

Reasonable precautions might include:

- making arrangements for easy access to a telephone if the house does not have one
- taking a second midwife with her
- alerting the hospital that the high-risk woman is now in labour
- informing the hospital of the woman's blood group prior to the birth to ensure it has supplies available
- taking with her an IV infusion and plasma
- having a qualified medical practitioner also attend the birth
- taking resuscitation equipment for the baby.

A midwife cannot be sued for negligence merely because she

attended a high-risk case at home. It would have to be demonstrated that she *acted* negligently or that her procedures were negligent. Having taken the actions suggested above it would be difficult to prove that she had not taken reasonable precautions.

Any mother who is informed that she is a high-risk case should check with a midwife, the Association for Improvements in the Maternity Services or the Society to Support Home Confinement to establish whether or not this diagnosis is correct. It is their experience that some mothers are told that they are high risk when they are not. This often occurs in areas where the Health Authority has a policy of 100 per cent hospital birth and wishes to prevent women having their babies at home. An incorrect diagnosis of high risk is a serious issue, as the anxiety caused by such a diagnosis may cause the mother increased stress and lead to unnecessary interventions.

Some common definitions of high risk:

- previous forceps delivery
- women under the age of 23 or over the age of 27 (only five years of low risk!)
- women expecting their first baby
- women expecting their third or more baby
- previous complicated birth
- high blood pressure
- previous retained placenta.

Any women given any of these reasons for not having a home birth should check with another midwife, AIMS or the Society to Support Home Confinement. For example, AIMS was approached by a woman who was told that she had high blood pressure and could not give birth at home. When she asked what the blood pressure was, she was told that it was 100/75. AIMS told her this was normal and the midwife was deliberately misleading her. It is not uncommon for women to find that their bp rises when they visit antenatal clinics. If this has happened to you ask for the midwife to visit your home and have your bp taken there.

CONSULTANT OPINION OR APPROVAL

Women wanting home births are often told that they have to see the consultant to check that they are able to have a home birth. This is unnecessary, and the interview has been used by many obstetricians as a means of persuading women to accept a hospital birth, often by 'shroud-waving', that is, telling them that they are irresponsible and that such action will cause the death of their babies.

A woman has every right to refuse to see the consultant. If, however, she feels that she ought to see him/her and she feels that s/he will not be sympathetic to what she wants to do she can safeguard herself by writing a letter to the consultant along the following lines:

Dear Mr/Ms
I have an appointment to see you on the . . . (insert date) to check that I am fit and healthy and that there are no complications.
   I have agreed to this appointment because I am concerned to ensure that my baby has the best possible care and attention. I am not, however, prepared to discuss my decision to have my baby at home and any attempt to raise this matter will be viewed by me as intimidation and I shall terminate the interview immediately and leave.

You should also ensure that you have someone with you at this appointment. Some women find such interviews stressful and need someone with them to give them support. It is unwise to attend on your own.

MIDWIVES

The majority of midwives are kind, considerate and caring people who are poorly paid, undervalued and often grossly overworked. There are, however, occasions when a woman may find herself with a midwife to whom she finds it difficult to relate.
   Should you find yourself in this position, do not ignore it, in the hope that the relationship might improve; take early action. It is difficult while concentrating on your labour to take action and dismiss the midwife!
   In this situation, the woman should consider writing to the Supervisor of Midwives informing her that she no longer wishes to be attended by this particular midwife and asking her to take steps to provide another. It should not be forgotten that a woman has an absolute right to refuse to be attended by any individual. Many mothers have successfully used this tactic when they wanted a particular midwife to attend them but have been told it was not possible. They have resolutely refused attendance from any other midwife and have written to the Supervisor of Midwives telling her that they will continue to do so unless they are attended by midwife X. This tactic can only be successful if the midwife the mother wants is willing to attend. It can happen that a midwife is happy to attend but the bureaucracy will not allow her. By stating clearly what you will or will not accept you can take the pressure

off the midwife and force the health authority to comply with your wishes.

If you call a midwife when you are in labour she has a legal duty to attend. She has to come and cannot refuse.

MIDWIFE REFERRALS

Some midwives have found that obstetricians have refused to accept a woman for a specific test (ultrasound, special blood test) on the grounds that the midwife must refer the woman through a GP. A midwife is an independent practitioner in her own right and she does not require the services of a GP for patient referrals. If an obstetrician blocks a midwife's referral you should complain to the District General Manager, with a copy to the Royal College of Midwives and the Association for Improvements in the Maternity Services. The latter organisation will be particularly interested and will help with any complaint you, or the midwife, may wish to make.

EMERGENCY HOSPITAL ADMISSION

There are some very rare occasions when a problem arises during a home birth and the midwife will need to take you into hospital. Having discussed her reasons for recommending a transfer to hospital, and having obtained your agreement, she will then contact the 'flying squad' (the emergency obstetric unit) and ask them to bring you into hospital.

By agreeing to a hospital admission you do not waive your right to be consulted about the proposed treatment. Furthermore, a hospital admission does not depend upon your agreeing to whatever they wish to do. In a recent case a midwife transferred a woman to hospital because when four centimetres dilated she had a hindwater leak which was heavily stained with meconium (a dark tarry substance from the baby's bowel, which usually indicates that the baby may be distressed). When they arrived at the hospital, the obstetrician refused to admit the woman unless she agreed to artificial rupture of the membranes and the attaching of a foetal scalp electrode to the baby's head. The mother did not want this, but agreed because she understood that she would not be admitted unless she did.

After the birth the midwife complained about the consultant's high handed actions and received clarification from the Regional Legal Adviser:

> The Health Authority has an obligation to provide maternity care and is bound to accept and care for any emergency when

asked to do so. . . . In these circumstances where a clinician feels that she cannot care for a particular individual, it will be for the hospital to find another doctor who will be willing to do so. Certainly there can be no question of any doctor turning a patient away from a hospital.

GP COVER FOR A HOME BIRTH

Some GPs refuse to attend home births and suggest to mothers that they seek another GP to provide cover. This is a waste of time. You should apply directly to the Supervisor of Midwives to book a home birth. If the midwives decide that the GP cover is necessary they have to arrange it, it has nothing to do with you and is not your responsibility.

STRIKING A WOMAN OR FAMILY OFF THE GP'S LIST

Many women have found that asking for a home birth has resulted in their being struck off by the GP. Some GPs even carry it to the extreme of striking off the whole family. If you have already signed an FP 24 (in Scotland, form D10) for maternity care with your GP, s/he cannot strike you off without your permission or without first approaching the FHSA (Scotland: Primary Care Division of the Health Board; Northern Ireland: Central Services Agency). If s/he has not sought your permission, you have grounds for complaining to the FHSA that s/he has broken her/his contract. You will need to make the complaint within thirteen weeks of being struck off (six weeks in Scotland, although the Scots are reconsidering their time limit).

It was generally believed that GPs took this action because they were particularly bloody-minded individuals. Recently, however, AIMS was approached by a midwife who had been told that the GP had struck a woman off his list because the Medical Defence Union (MDU) had advised him that 'I am still responsible for the birth of one of my patients. Even though I have declined to be involved I am still responsible and the only way I can get out of this responsibility is to strike Mrs X off my list.'

AIMS challenged the Medical Defence Union to identify the legal basis for this piece of advice. They were unable to do so. If you have been stuck off by your GP for daring to ask for a home birth you could ask him/her why s/he has taken such action. If it has been done on the advice of the MDU, you could draw his/her attention to the above and suggested that s/he re-consider.

DISPOSAL OF THE PLACENTA

Following the birth of a baby at home the midwife usually takes the placenta with her for disposal (the Health Authority usually sells it). It is, however, the mother's property and she may, if she wishes, keep it (even when she has given birth in hospital). Some couples like to ceremoniously bury it in the garden! Others decide to eat it! Apparently it tastes like liver.

One woman who suffered severe postnatal depression with her first pregnancy decided to eat her placenta raw. She kept it in the freezer and each day sliced off a small piece and ate it. She had no postnatal depression and believes that the hormones in the placenta helped maintain a balance during the early postnatal period and prevented postnatal depression on this occasion. It would be interesting to conduct a randomised controlled trial to see if this initiative works with other women.

6

CHOOSING A HOSPITAL BIRTH

The practice of delivering nearly all babies in hospital has contributed to the dramatic reduction in stillbirths and neonatal deaths and to the avoidance of many child handicaps ('Maternity Care in Action', 1984).
There is no evidence to support the claim that the safest policy is for all women to give birth in hospital (Rona Campbell and Alison Macfarlane, 1989).

Choosing where to give birth to your baby is one of the most important and significant decisions you will ever make. If you are a low-risk, fit and healthy woman, who wants to have a normal birth, then apart from a GP unit, a hospital (particularly a consultant unit, teaching hospital or private maternity unit) will be the one place where you will stand the least chance of achieving what you want.

The confidence of many women in their ability to give birth normally has been seriously undermined by continuous references to the dangers of giving birth outside a hospital and, as a result, many women are still willing to take the added risk of having a baby in hospital in the misguided belief that this is the safest place to give birth.

As Marjorie Tew has clearly exposed in her excellent book *Safer Childbirth?* not only does the research evidence show that giving birth under consultant care *increase* the risks of death and morbidity for the mother and child, but that over the years obstetricians have deliberately misinterpreted the evidence and concealed the facts. Primarily to further the interests of their own professional control of childbirth. Something which they are still doing today.

As Tew revealed, each year over 2,400 babies die as a *direct result* of a hospital booking. Had those women booked into GP units or stayed at home those deaths could have been avoided.

There are a variety of maternity units around the country, but you may not have the full range within your area. You should, however, find out which ones you do have:

- teaching hospital
- consultant unit
- general practitioner unit
- general practitioner unit within a consultant unit
- general practitioner beds within a consultant unit
- private hospitals.

If you do decide that you wish to have your baby in the nearest obstetric unit or teaching hospital, there are steps that you can take to limit the amount of interference that is common in many of these units.

The majority of maternity units will claim that they do not use technology routinely but 'only when there are indications'. Unfortunately the indications are so numerous that the majority of women suffer them. The only way that you can deal with this, (and as a by-product discover the true risks of birth in a particular unit) is to find out about their statistics. Your first approach should be to the hospital; you can ask it to provide annual figures for the previous two years for the following:

- total number of babies born
- total number of maternities (mothers giving birth)
- average number of ultrasound scans per pregnancy (one)
- artificial rupture of membranes (breaking the waters) (Less than 10 per cent).
- induction of labour (by oxytocin drip or vaginal pessary)
- acceleration of Labour (by oxytocin drip)
- epidural anaesthesia (spinal anaesthetic to block sensation in the lower body) (less than 10 per cent)
- other drugs during labour (such as pethidine, sedatives etc.)
- electronic foetal monitoring (monitor attached to the baby's scalp or a buckle across the mother's stomach).
- forceps delivery
- ventouse delivery (vacuum extraction using suction cup attached to the baby's head)
- Caesarean operations (less than 10 per cent)
- episiotomies (cut made to enlarge the vaginal entrance) (less than 15 per cent).
- number of babies admitted to intensive or special care baby unit

• number of babies receiving Vitamin K injection (Less than 10 per cent).

Note: As a general rule of thumb each of the procedures quoted above should not exceed 20 per cent of the total number of maternities, except in those instances where a lower figure has been quoted.

An alternative approach is to contact your local National Child-birth Trust group and ask them if they have any statistics about local births. They may only have details of the birth experiences of the women who have been through NCT classes. In which case remember that women attending NCT classes are generally *low* risk, and should therefore have *very* few interventions. If they have a high levels of intervention (i.e. greater than those figures suggested in the above list) then you can be sure that too much interference is occurring in that unit.

Many hospitals will refuse to release their statistics, in that case you should approach your Community Health Council (Scotland: Local Health Council; Northern Ireland: District Committee). Some CHCs will be reluctant to obtain the figures, but any good CHC should already have them in order to evaluate the quality of local services. Otherwise how can they be effective as the users' 'watch-dog'?

Community Health Councils have a statutory right to obtain hospital statitics; if they seem reluctant you can point out to them that as they are supposed to represent local service users they should be obtaining these statistics for you. Don't, however, expect them to produce the results quickly, it does take some time. If they persist in their refusal, attend the public session of their meeting (they usually meet once a month) and ask for the statistics publicly. If they still refuse, try contacting the local press. You can make sure the press attends by telephoning the local paper before the meeting and telling them what you propose to do.

The usual response from most hospitals to requests for infor-mation about procedures is to suggest that they do nothing routinely, but only when indicated. What they omit to mention is that they usually have very high levels of 'indication'.

If the figures you receive exceed those suggested in the above list in a number of categories, you should consider changing hospitals or making a booking which will give you a greater chance of having as near a normal delivery as it is possible to get in a hospital. For instance, you could book a domino birth (see p. 57) which will provide care from a community midwife and will give you a better chance of having a normal birth.

Choice of hospital birth:

- consultant care
- shared care
- domino birth
- 6- or 48-hour discharge
- private care

CONSULTANT CARE

Consultant obstetricians are experts in abnormality and obviously provide essential expertise for the few cases of high-risk births, but over the years they have taken over the care of normal birth and amended it to fit their own perceptions. The majority has little contact, either during their training or in their later appointments, with normal pregnancies and births. This results in an attitude that childbirth is essentially an illness which is best 'cured' by hospital care and technological interventions. They have little faith and even less understanding of the importance of the confidence of the mother and the subtle negative influences of standard hospital procedures.

What occurs is an attitude which is best described as the 'just-in-case syndrome'. Just-in-case you get an infection, you have pubic shaving. Just-in-case your labour doesn't progress you will be induced. Just-in-case your baby has problems you will have electronic foetal monitoring. Just-in-case the pain is too much you will have drugs. Just-in-case the baby is distressed you will have an episiotomy. Such attitudes create anxieties in the labour wards and result in an over-use of obstetric technology, much of which was developed to help mothers and babies with real problems but is often used routinely on mothers who do not have any – until they suffer unnecessary interventions.

SHARED CARE

Shared care is a system where you usually receive your antenatal care from your GP and/or midwife in your community but come into hospital for the birth. Usually you will be asked to visit the hospital for some of your antenatal appointments. The system varies a great deal throughout the country. Some women have found that instead of reducing the number of antenatal appointments it actually increased them, they had antenatal care from their GP and this was repeated at the hospital.

In some shared-care schemes the mother carries her own case notes. In spite of the fact that this has been done successfully in a number of areas for many years the proposal has been met with suspicion and anxiety by some members of the hospital staff. They felt that giving women their case notes would result in the notes being lost; they were also very anxious about women reading what the staff had written about them.

Research has shown that giving women the case notes improved the quality of care and encouraged women to become more involved with their care; because they could read the case notes they could point out any inaccuracies. It reduced the practice of writing libellous and incorrect statements about the women in the notes and also resulted in fewer case notes being lost. Over a two-year period one hospital found that none of the case notes had been lost, whereas in the previous system at least two case notes a week went missing.

DOMINO BIRTH

A 'domino' birth is derived from the rather cumbersome explanation *dom*iciliary midwifery *in* and *out* — hence domino. It means that you will be cared for by your local midwife both in and out of hospital. She will look after you antenatally, sometimes independently, sometimes with your GP. She will give you your antenatal care and once you go into labour she will visit your home and examine you. She will decide when to transfer you to hospital where she will help you give birth to your baby, tidy up and then (usually after a couple of hours) take you home again. She will then look after you and your baby for the statutory ten days following the birth.

Many women like this scheme because it means that they have their care from a midwife they know and the decision to go into hospital rests with the midwife, thus avoiding the error so many women make in arriving in hospital too early. In some areas, however, women are told to go to the hospital when they go into labour, and either their own midwife is called in (a decision which is made by the hospital staff) or the woman is looked after by the hospital staff and is allowed to go home six hours, or so, after the birth. This system is *not* a domino delivery.

Sometimes, women have been told that they cannot go home until the afternoon because they have not been 'passed as fit' and must wait for the doctor's rounds. Or they have been told that they could not go home because the ambulances were all busy and the hospital would not accept them being discharged to their own private transport. A woman can discharge herself, and her baby, from hospital at any time and does not need the consent of the doctors or midwives. She is not obliged to return home in an ambulance and may use her own private transport if she wishes, or be taken home in the midwife's car.

Any woman booking a domino delivery should make sure that

she will be allocated a local midwife and that the midwife, or her colleague will attend her in the manner described in the first paragraph.

Should your local midwife appear unwilling, or unable, to provide a domino booking you can insist upon this type of booking. Write to the Supervisor of Midwives asking her to make the necessary arrangements.

Women are often asked to attend the hospital antenatal clinic in the usual way. Though not a true domino booking, it is fine if the arrangement suits you. If it does not, you can insist on receiving your antenatal care at home or your GP/midwives' clinic.

Should your circumstances change, or you wish to change to a standard hospital booking or a home-birth booking, you should first of all notify your community midwife of your wish to change and she will make the necessary alterations. It will be unlikely for the midwife not to take action on a request for a change to a standard hospital booking, as the bureaucracy is only too keen to book women into hospital. You may find, however, that the midwife is not happy to change your booking to a home birth. If that is so, you should write a letter to the Supervisor of Midwives saying that you intend having a home birth and intend cancelling your previous booking. The letter could be on the lines of the letter to the Supervisor of Midwives contained in the home-birth section (see page 44).

In many areas there is a very serious shortage of midwives, and many women are told that there are insufficient staff to offer a domino scheme. Improvements in maternity care will not be achieved unless women demand what they want and what they believe is important. If a domino birth is what you want, do not be persuaded otherwise. The staffing problems will never be solved by persuading women to put up with a form of care they don't want, don't like and yet feel obliged to use.

6- OR 48-HOUR DISCHARGE

If you want to stay in hospital for as short a time as possible, you can ask for one of these bookings. It will mean that you will have whatever kind of antenatal care you want to arrange, but you will go into hospital and be delivered by a hospital midwife and come home shortly afterwards. This system is not to be confused with a domino birth. To have a domino you will have to be taken in by your own community midwife. In some areas midwives try to persuade mothers that the 6 -or 48-hour discharge is the same as a domino; it is not.

7

CHOOSING PRIVATE CARE

The National Health Services was established in order to ensure that free health care was available at the time of need. The expansion of private hospitals and the involvement of doctors in private care results in a continuing decline in the standards of service within the NHS: private hospitals milk the profitable side of the service, and leaving the unprofitable to decline. The controls on private care are also minimal. Many small private maternity units would not be allowed to function were they within the NHS; but not only is it difficult to obtain statistics from these units, there is also an official reluctance to monitor them.

Choosing private maternity care does not necessarily ensure that you have an obstetrician attending your delivery nor does it mean that you will have a safer birth. On the contrary, private maternity units have the highest infant mortality rates, the highest morbidity rates and higher levels of litigation than any other area of maternity care. Private units do, however, provide excellent hotel facilities. You will have your own private room, good food, and often a bottle of champagne provided following the birth.

PRIVATE HOSPITALS

It is possible to book care with your consultant privately and have your baby in a private hospital. Martin Richards in an article about obstetric practice (1979) stated that there was strong suggestive evidence that perinantal mortality and morbidity are higher for private patients than for comparable women delivered within the NHS (see page 157). The reasons for this are not fully explained, mainly because of the lack of statistical information from private care. The majority of patients going into private care are usually women from the wealthier social groups and therefore fitter and healthier than the majority of the population. One explanation may be that women having private care generally have more interventions than other groups, more inductions, more drugs etc.

If you book privately, and you want a consultant to deliver you, he will more than likely suggest that you come in for an induction on a specific day in order to fit in with his other commitments. The induction is more likely to be suggested because it is convenient for him, rather than because your baby needs to be induced on that day.

You can check by finding out whether or not any mothers are due to be induced on that day. You can also find out whether that particular day of the week is the usual day when Mr X does his inductions.

Medical insurance companies pay out more money if an intervention has been carried out (they do not increase their payments for normal deliveries). Unfortunately, private care units are not required to produce statistics of their practice and it is, therefore, very difficult to assess the quality of the care they are offering.

One serious drawback with private hospitals is that should you be dissatisfied with your care, apart from not paying your bill, you have no channel of complaint. The NHS, for all its faults, has a complaints system and a means of checking on all complaints. This does not exist with private maternity units. Furthermore, many private maternity units have few facilities for dealing with an emergency; if you are considering booking into a private unit ask if there is a resident anaesthetist and what provision they have for dealing with an obstetric emergency.

PRIVATE MIDWIVES

A midwife is an indepedent practitioner in her own right and she can if she wishes undertake private work, and advertise. All private midwives do home births and they provide a full service during your pregnancy, birth and antenatally for around £1,000.

Private midwives usually practise in this way because they have become very dissatisfied with the quality of service they were giving women within the NHS. All private midwives give continuity of care; they sometimes work in small groups of two or three, so you will only have a small number of women to get to know during your pregnancy; and they actively support and encourage normal physiological childbirth (many of them use homoeopathic remedies as well as the usual drugs that are available during pregnancy and labour).

The majority of private midwives are in London, but there are others around the country. They can be contacted through the Independent Midwives' Association, 65 Mount Nod Road, London SW16 2LP or Special Delivery, 34 Elm Quay Court, Nine Elms Lane, London SW8 5DE, 071 498 2322.

8

GENERAL ISSUES

AMENITY BEDS

If you would prefer to have a room of your own you can ask for an amenity bed. Not all hospitals have them and those that do will charge a small fee for each day you are in the room. In most hospitals amenity beds are allocated on the understanding that if an emergency occurs and they require the room then you will move out to an ordinary ward.

COMPANION IN LABOUR

The Short Report recommended that women should be able to choose up to two people to accompany her in labour. There is, however, no legal obligation for the hospital to agree to the Short Report's suggestion. Although it is now generally accepted that the father or a companion can stay with the mother, in some hospitals the staff still employ subtle tactics to get them out of the way. 'Why don't you go home and get some rest, your wife will be a long time yet, and we will ring you as soon as anything starts.' They then omit to ring until the last moment.

At Plymouth General Hospital a woman complained that she had spent hours pleading with the staff to telephone her husband; they rang so late he arrived just in time to see her wheeled into theatre for a caesarean section. In their reply the hospital stated, 'She asked for him to be called at 2200 hours on the night she delivered but the staff felt that she wasn't in established labour and that it was too early.'

The opinions of the staff are irrelevant. The mother instructed them to contact her husband because she felt she needed him.

They deliberately ignored her instructions and, what was worse, the midwife's inaction was supported by the senior staff in the correspondence that followed. So much for a hospital which advertises itself as being responsive to parents' wishes.

CONSENT TO TREATMENT

The Medical Defence Union Booklet *Consent to Treatment* (1974) contained the following entry on maternity patients:

> The Union does not consider that a maternity patient need give her written consent to any operative or manipulative procedure that is normally associated with childbirth. When she enters hospital for her confinement it can be assumed that she assents to any necessary procedure, including the administration of a local, general or other anaesthetic.

This statement was challenged by AIMS, which was informed by its legal advisors that they did not believe that this statement would stand up in a court of law. After AIMS drew attention to this in their booklet *Denial of Parents' Rights in Childbirth* the Medical Defence Union withdrew the statement from the next edition of their booklet.

In common law, any doctor of midwife giving treatment which the mother has refused leaves him/herself open to a charge of assault. Any mother given treatment against her wishes, after she has refused, should make an immediate complaint to the District General Manager, c/o the hospital, and immediately contact AIMS, Health Rights (if they are in London) or Action for Victims of Medical Accidents.

MALE MIDWIVES

All midwifery training schools have now to accept male midwives if they apply for training. The staff should make it clear to you, before you go into hospital, that you might be attended by a male midwife and that you may decide whether or not you wish to be attended by them.

You have an absolute right to refuse to be attended by a male midwife (or a male doctor for that matter) if you wish. You can make it clear before you go into hospital by adding your consent or refusal your letter to the hospital.

MEDICAL AND MIDWIFERY STUDENTS

A mother who does not wish to be attended by a medical or midwifery student has the right to refuse; she can also refuse to admit medical/midwifery students to the labour suite while she is in labour or giving birth.

Obviously, both medical and midwifery students need training and you may feel that you would like to help with that. In which case you could insist that if a medical or midwifery student is going to be present for the birth of your baby that they attend you throughout your labour.

One of the problems with medical student training is that students are indoctrinated with the attitude that birth is very dangerous and anything can go wrong without warning at any time. This is reinforced by their being called in a rush to 'an interesting delivery' – twins, breech, etc. They rarely have the chance to see a labour all the way through and, therefore, often fail to understand what normality is all about.

One other point to bear in mind with being attended by students is that you stand a higher chance of having a routine episiotomy with a student present (they have to learn how to do them); you have the right to refuse an episiotomy if you feel it is being done more for training than real need.

The following is a fairly typical example of the information given to parents (at a Glasgow hospital) about their right to refuse to be attended by a medical student (no mention of midwifery students):

Teaching of medical students
Medical students receive some of their training at Rutherglen Maternity Hospital and may be present at your consultation. We are sure that you will appreciate the need for students to be taught and to gain practical experience and that you will not mind their presence. *If you do mind*, please make this known to the doctor or nurse who will ensure that your wishes are followed.

This kind of form is unacceptable because it applies subtle pressure to encourage the women to comply. Instead of being offered the choice of equally weighted options it is subtly suggested that you would not mind. You then have to opt out. This pressure combined with that of a woman being surrounded by people who want her to agree will often be enough to ensure reluctant compliance.

An acceptable form would say:

Teaching of medical or midwifery students
This hospital provides training for medical and midwifery students. During your visits and stay here you may be approach- ed by them for permission to attend a consultation or to be involved in your care, for example, delivering your baby under

supervision. You may agree or refuse. The decision is entirely yours and your future care will in no way be affected by the decision you choose to make. If you wish you may ask for your decision to be recorded in your case notes.

If you are going into a unit which you know has medical or midwifery students you need to think about your views beforehand, some of the things you may wish to consider will be. Would you be happy or unhappy:

• with one student being present?
• with more than one student?
• if the student was male or female?
• if the student was a midwifery student?
• if the student was a medical student?
• for the student to be present for an antenatal appointment?
• for the student to be present all the way through your labour?
• if the student was called in just for the delivery?

Having thought about what or would would not be acceptable to you you can tell anybody involved with your care of your decision. If you have made a birth plan you can draw their attention to your statement there. If you do not have a birth plan, or the hospitals' birth plan does not include this in their selected choices, you can inform them of your decision and ask for it to be entered into your case notes.

If you are reluctant to make these views known yourself you could ask your partner, relative, or friend to make them for you.

FLYING SQUADS (THE EMERGENCY OBSTETRIC UNIT)

The first 'flying squad' or emergency obstetric unit was set up in Bellshill, Lanarkshire, in 1933. The aim was to give expert emergency care to women too ill or too shocked to be moved to hospital without preliminary treatment. With the move to 'encourage' all women into hospital there have been constant moves to disband this service.

In 1961 a survey of flying squads showed that 60 per cent of calls were for third-stage problems. By 1976 an examination of flying squad calls at St Thomas's Hospital in London showed that out of twenty-five calls, only four were justified (two ante-partum haemorrhages, one retained placenta and one retained products of conception, and a further three calls might have been justified (one post-partum and two ante-partum haemorrhages). The proportion of third-stage problems was only 20 per cent. From this study is was concluded that 'few, if any, circumstances in modern obstetric practice merit continuing the flying squad in the urban area'. Most patients would have done as well or better by going straight to hospital in an ordinary ambulance.

In 1980 a midwife, Janet Jennings, was attending, at home, a young pregnant woman who was bleeding. The day before a colleague had called the flying squad and they had taken one and a half hours to arrive, so in view of this, and her own personal experiences of the inadequacy of the flying squad, Janet decided to take the woman into hospital herself. Within fifty-five minutes of receiving the original call the woman was in hospital receiving appropriate care. The Superviser of Midwives reported her to the Central Midwives Board (the predecessor of the English National Board), who subsequently reprimanded her for failing to call a flying squad. Had she called the flying squad, with their track record, the woman would probably have died.

In September 1988 another midwife, Jilly Rosser, was struck off for misconduct after she took a mother and new-born baby about two-thirds of a mile to hospital, in her car, instead of waiting for an ambulance. It was in the same area as Janet Jennings practised, and over the years the Health Authority had done nothing to improve the flying squad facilities.

Jilly was subsequently re-instated but these cases have resulted in many midwives feeling very unsupported when they attend a home birth. Since that time consultant obstetricians have continued trumpeting their opinion that all women should have their babies in hospital, despite there being *no evidence* that this kind of care is beneficial for all women and babies.

Every Health Authority now has shortages of midwifery staff, and in some areas this shortage is serious. One of the solutions to this problem has been the attempt to completely withdraw the home-birth service and disband the flying squads, suggesting instead that women dial 999 and they will be taken to hospital by ambulance. This arrangement is unsatisfactory, ambulancemen have only a few hours midwifery training and no obstetric training. This system puts all women at unnecessary risk and you should be checking that your health authority is not relying on such a service. If they are, inform AIMS.

Ironically, one of the greatest risks women run is a post-partum haemorrhage following the use of oxytocin for induction or acceleration of labour. A study in Southampton showed that women who have oxytocin run twice the risk of a post-partum haemorrhage for up to ten days post-natally, than those women who have not had oxytocin.

Now that hospitals 'encourage' women to go home as soon as possible, in some cases after six hours, it is those women who will need a flying squad service. Yet, more and more, areas are withdrawing this service.

In February 1988 the Court of Appeal decided that a health authority was liable for the negligent organisation and delivery of maternity services when they failed to provide a consultant or registrar to attend a twin delivery, in a consultant unit, which ran into problems. It may be that it is time that someone took a Health Authority to court for negligently failing to provide an adequate emergency obstetric unit. But before we do that we have to find out just how bad the services are in some areas, and hold some discussions to find out what reasonable alternatives there might be.

9

BIRTH PLANS

The majority of women express the view that they would like to have a normal birth, and the majority of them will have 'normal' delivery written on their case notes. But what is normal?

It would not be unreasonable to define a normal birth as a birth which follows a physiological course without interventions which would pervert it. Hospital midwives and doctors describe a normal delivery as any vaginal birth which does not involve the use of forceps or ventouse. So it is possible to go into hospital, have your waters broken, a foetal scalp electrode screwed into your baby's scalp, an oxytocin drip inserted, an epidural anaesthetic and an episiotomy and be described as having had a normal delivery.

Any woman experiencing any one or a combination of the above should not consider that she has had a normal birth. It is this confusion which leads women into believing that childbirth is a dreadful, painful and excruciating experience through which they have to go in order to have a baby.

Normal childbirth in Britain has been so perverted by routine hospital practices that the majority of women have no idea of what normal birth is. Those who have experienced a normal birth and a technological birth can testify to how different the two experiences are.

Many women seem to believe that they can order a normal birth rather like ordering a leg of lamb from the butchers. Unfortunately, life is not like that. If you want to have a normal labour and birth you will have to do your homework, and you will need to understand what helps a normal birth and what works against it. There is a wide variety of childbirth books and magazines available and a number of childbirth organisations which give help and advice.

You can read the books and contact the organisations.

Many women believe that writing a birth plan will help them get the kind of birth they want. This is possible, but it will also depend on the kind of birth attendant you have. Getting a good, sympathetic, midwife (particularly in a teaching hospital or consultant unit) depends to a great extent on the luck of the draw. If you are going to make sure that the cards are stacked in your favour then you will have to do your homework. Making out a birth plan is one possible step in the right direction.

The idea of birth plans evolved from 'A Letter to the Midwife', a document prepared by the Association of Radical Midwives in response to the growing anger of the user groups to the way in which hospitals responded to requests for alternative treatment. It was not uncommon for parents to arrange what they thought was an agreed birth plan – for instance, a Leboyer birth (where the lights are kept low, noise is reduced to a minimum and the baby is delivered in a gentle manner and given an immediate warm bath) or perhaps a squatting birth – only to find that the staff on duty ignored or overruled their wishes. The mother could refer any new midwife or doctor to the notes and if the hospital refused to put her letter in the notes she had time to find herself another hospital.

Since then, some hospitals have compiled their own birth plans and are offering them to mothers to fill in. The risk of that idea is that women may well be manipulated into agreeing to what the hospital wants to provide and, unless they are given information about the issues involved, can be easily drawn into a position where the hospital does as it pleases while giving the impression that it is responding to the parents' wishes.

The Huddersfield Birth plan

	Would like	No strong views	Wish to avoid
On admission in labour Partial shave Enema Presence of partner/relative/ friend Wearing own nightdress			

During labour
Continuous monitoring of
   baby's heart rate by
   electronic machine
Correcting a slow labour by
   rupture of the membranes
   (breaking the waters)
Correcting a slow labour by an
   intravenous infusion (drip)
Presence of partner/relative/
   friend			

Pain control Pethidine or other drugs by injection Gas and oxygen face mask Epidural			

Delivery
Presence of partner/
   relative/friend if normal
   delivery
Presence of partner/relative/
   friend if complications with
   delivery (eg forceps)
Episiotomy			

The birth plan was published in *Maternal and Child Health* as an example of a hospital's initiative in offering women their own birth plan. The aim was 'to make women well prepared for labour so that they can gain greater satisfaction from the event'. The women were asked to choose by putting a tick in the appropriate column.

The birth plan was not only interesting for its selection of choices but also for its lack of choice. Few mothes would question why partial pubic shaving and enemas are still being carried out yet research shows that pubic shaving *increases* infections and enemas are totally unncessary for the majority of women.

All the choices in the 'during labour' section involve technological interventions. Continuous electronic foetal monitoring increases the Caesarean section rate, is ineffective and uncomfortable and no definition of a 'slow labour' is given; nor are the women offered any alternatives for dealing with a slow labour other than drugs and rupturing the membranes.

The section on pain control only offers drugs. Pethidine is ineffective 70 per cent of the time, and epidurals increase the risk of forceps delivery, can cause breathing difficulties for the baby at birth and increase the risk of Caesarean sections.

For the delivery, many parents might like to choose the position they give birth in. They may wish to decide whether or not to have syntometrine, or a multitude of other choices, yet the hospital only offers them the choice of having a partner present and deciding whether or not have an episiotomy. Interestingly, 6 per cent of women chose to have an episiotomy, primarily because of fears of excessive tearing at the delivery. One wonders how many of those women would have made that choice had they been informed that episiotomy makes no difference at all to the risk of tearing and for some their sex lives will be affected for longer than those women who delivered normally or who had a tear.

If birth plans are going to be used by hospitals then they must be accompanied by some notes about the procedures that are listed, and advice on where the women can find additional information if they want. It is all very well a woman 'choosing' to have an episiotomy, but was her choice an informed one? What kind of choice would she have made if she was aware of the benefits and risks of this procedure? Supporting whatever the parents want when their choices are made without full information is as bad as dictating to women what kind of care they must have because of hospital policy. It is fine for a woman to make a choice to have an episiotomy after she has had information about its benefits and risks, but to ask her to tick a box of carefully selected 'options' is simply an exercise in public relations. It merely gives her the illusion of being involved in the decision-making process.

YOUR BIRTH PLAN

Once you have sorted out *where* you want to have your baby you can concentrate on informing the midwives of the *kind* of birth you want. You could ask for an interview with the Supervisor of Midwives or even your obstetrician (though he may not feel inclined to see you) to discuss this. You should take your partner with you and have your questions written down. It is worth knowing that doctors and midwives work in teams and that different teams may have different policies according to which consultant is in charge. Try to find out if there are any differences in approach and policies so that you can choose the most sympathetic team.

There are hospitals which will be very reluctant to tell you about their policies, using a favourite expression 'we do not use routine procedures here, we only intervene when necessary'. If you particularly want a natural birth, then it is important to apreciate that obstetricians, on the whole, are sceptical about them. Partly because they meet so few women who achieve it, and partly because they'd be out of a job if too many women succeeded!

Make it clear that you are not challenging the quality of their obstetric care and that, of course, you will accept drugs or other forms of intervention if you and the obstetrician agree that it is absolutely necessary for the safety and comfort of you or the baby. These are some of the points you might like to discuss:

- I would like my husband/partner/friend to be present throughout labour and birth.
  Note: Check that they will not be invited to leave for *any* reason. Stressful situations are the very times when a supportive companion is needed. Research has shown that a supportive lay companion has significant effects on the labour: it is shorter, mothers were awake more after the delivery, and they stroke, smile and talk to their babies more than mothers who did not have a companion (Sosa, R. *et al*, 1980).
- I would like to know what their policy is with regard to induction/ acceleration (augmentation) of labour, and what methods are used.
  Note. You will need to find out what percentage of first-time mothers have this done (they are the ones who usually get higher levels of intervention). Ask your CHC for the figures. If they are over 20 per cent, when combined then it is likely that these procedures are being done routinely.
- I do not want to have my waters broken on admission.
  Note: This is a routine in many hospitals and results in the staff being committed to delivery within a certain time because of the

potential problems of infection following the internal examinations. This can sometimes lead to a Caesarean section because
of lack of progress. Studies have shown that there is a greater risk
of infection *if frequent internal examinations are made.*

- I do not want my pubic hair shaved.
  Note: If you have a lush forest of pubic hair and you need
  stitching the midwife may well wish to clip your hair with
  scissors since the last thing you want is your hair tangled up with
  the stitches! Research has shown that shaving pubic hair has no
  benefit whatsoever and increases discomfort and itching as the
  hair regrows. The researchers concluded that 'perineal shaving is
  an unjustified assault and should be abandoned' (Romney, M.
  et al, 1980).

- I do not want to be given an enema, unless it can be shown that I
  have an impacted bowel (constipated).
  Note: Research has shown that giving women enemas does not
  prevent faecal contamination during the labour: 'Enemas should
  be reserved for women who have not had their bowels open in
  the past twenty-four hours and have an obviously loaded rectum
  on initial pelvic examination' (Romney, M. *et al*, 1981).

- I do not want to be given any pain-killing drugs unless and until
  I ask for them.

- I would prefer not to have any form of medical interference
  unless it is explained to me that it is absolutely necessary. If
  labour is proceeding without complication I do not want to have
  any form of electronic foetal monitoring (which restricts you to
  lying on your back, a position that is of little benefit to the baby
  and can *cause* foetal distress).

- I would like to be able to move around freely during labour and
  give birth in a position that is comfortable for me.

- I do not want to be given an episiotomy unless absolutely
  necessary. Should it become necessary to carry out an episiotomy
  I do not agree to being stitched by a medical student.
  Note: It is not unknown, in many hospitals, for stitching to be
  carried out by a student who has never before done any kind of
  stitching — in other words students are practising stitching on
  the most sensitive part of a woman's anatomy'

- I would prefer the baby not to be born under bright lights with a
  lot of noise; I would like my baby to be handled gently and to be
  given me immediately and for as long as possible; I would prefer
  the staff to wait until the cord has stopped pulsating before they
  cut it; I would prefer the baby's mucus not be sucked out
  (routine gastric suctioning) unless necessary.
  Note: There is no justification for routine gastric suctioning in
  the delivery room, the research shows that this is a practice

which should be abandoned (see Enkin, M., Keirse, M. and Chalmers, I., 1989). You have the right to refuse to have it done. If the mother has been given syntometrine or ergometrine the midwife (or obstetrician) has to decide between clamping the cord immediately the baby is born, thereby denying him/her the extra physiological quota of 90ml (3oz) of blood; or alternatively, leaving the cord and risking the possibility of the baby becoming overtransfused as blood is forced into the baby by the energetic contractions of the uterus (Inchy, S., 1982).

• If for any reason my baby has to be separated from me (for example, to be taken into special care) I would like to be able to go with my baby and be able to give my child breast-milk.
Note: Research shows that there is no justification for separating mothers and babies for observation (Inchy, S., 1982). If you would like to breast feed it is important that it takes place as soon after birth as you and the baby want, and that you state that you do not wish your child to be given any bottles, for any reason, or to be taken into a nursery.

• I would like my husband/partner/friend and myself to have time alone together with the baby after the birth.

• I would like my other children, to be able to visit me as soon as possible after the birth and frequently thereafter.

• I am willing/not willing to be attended by a male midwife.

• I am not willing to be delivered by midwifery students or medical students unless those students have stayed with me from the beginning of my labour.
Note: Unfortunately, medical students rarely see the whole of a normal labour; consequently they have little idea of what it is like. The usual procedure is for the medical student (and some-times the midwifery student) to come in near delivery and deliver the baby. Such policies result in medical students having little idea of the progress of a normal labour. By insisting that you will only agree to be attended by students if they are with you throughout your labour you will help change the attitude that birth is a dangerous process and anything can happen at any time that is ingrained in the many medical minds.

• I do not agree to an ultrasound examination unless the infor-mation required cannot be obtained by other means.
Note: Research evidence shows that ultrasound increases the risk of pre-term labour, and there is some evidence which shows that ultrasound may cause dyslexia (problems with reading and writing) in some children who have been exposed in the womb to this procedure. Whilst uncertainty exists it is best to avoid routine ultrasound examinations if you can. If you do feel you need an ultrasound examination you can insist that the staff fill

in the ultrasound record form and insert it on your notes (Stark *et al*, 1984).

- In order to ensure that I have the best chance of having my wishes considered I would prefer to be attended by a midwife whom I have known throughout my pregnancy. In this way both she, and I, will know each other's views and I will be confident in any advice that she may wish to give me. I do, however, understand that this system of care is not yet available in all hospitals. If it is not available in yours then I will accept the arrangements that have been made but wish to record that I feel that it is not providing me with the best means of support.
- You may also wish to discuss the possibility of your baby being bathed after birth (for relaxing not cleansing purposes). Most important, do have someone with you during your labour who can help you to relax and explain what you want and need during labour.

Finally, you could add that the above list is an example of what you would *like* to happen during your birth. It may be that for various reasons you may change your mind, or it may be necessary to depart from what you would like. If that were to happen you would hope that the midwives would understand that such an option exists. You hope that your midwife will do her best to accommodate your wishes, just as you will do your best to listen to and discuss any recommendation she may wish to make.

This looks a daunting list of topics to be discussed – but just pick out the points that are most important to you. Get as much as you can written in your notes, so that if, during labour, you are unfortunate enough to have unsympathetic attendants, then you can refer them to your interview and the fact that certain things have been agreed.

Occasionally a woman will find herself attended by unsympathetic attendants. This need not be tolerated, you can refuse to be attended by them and insist that a replacement is found. Anyone giving treatment after the mother has refused risks being sued for assault.

If you find the thought of approaching anyone in hospital with a list of questions and requests too intimidating, don't despair. You could put your list into a letter form and send it to the Supervisor of Midwives at the hospital, asking for her comments.

Your letter could be on the following lines. (If you wish this letter can be written in the form of a joint letter and signed by both you and your husband/partner.)

Dear

I am expecting a baby sometime in . . . I would like to give
birth to my baby in hospital and I would appreciate it if you
would comment on your hospital's policy concerning the
following:

(You can then list the items you particularly want).

I do not consent to the following:

(You can then list the items you particularly do not want).

I have been careful to ensure that I am in good health and well
prepared for the birth. I am, therefore, most concerned to
ensure that I and my baby have the best birth experience
possible and for that reason I would like to be informed of
your hospital's policy on the items I have listed.

I would also like confirmation, should I book into your
hospital for the birth of my baby, that this letter would be
attached to my notes.

I shall look forward to your reply.

Yours sincerely

It is most important to examine closely the response you get from
the hospital. If you get a helpful response, be sure to ask for your
letter to attached to your file. If the letter does not really answer
your questions, or you are told that you can discuss your questions
with the staff when you come in to have the baby, that is the time
to consider finding yourself another hospital. If they will not put
their policies into writing, or are not prepared to include the letter
with your case notes, then that is a hospital which is unlikely to pay
much attention to your wishes once you get in there.

If you have already considered the kind of treatment you want,
and the kind of treatment you do not want, a great deal can be
done when you are in labour – providing you and your partner are
prepared. Many people have got the sort of birth they wanted by
refusing unnecessary interventions and by telling their medical
attendants at the time.

Unfortunately, there are still hospitals which remove babies from
their mothers and put them into nurseries at night. No one has the
right to remove your baby against your wishes; just firmly tell the
staff that you intend keeping your baby with you *all the time* and
that since you are breast-feeding immediately on demand, your
baby will not disturb anyone else.

Be clear about what you want; be firm and straightforward; try not to be aggressive; remember, no one has the right to do anything to you or your baby without your permission. Be prepared, but above all remember that your attitude and your love towards your baby are what matter most — not whether you manage to achieve the 'perfect' birth.

When approaching staff with your proposals, or at any time during your pregnancy and birth, remember that the vast majority of midwives are very nice people. They do their job under enormous pressures and strains and try their best to respond to your wishes. Unfortunately, the midwives often find themselves being bashed from both directions; from the users who want a good birth and from their colleagues and the bureaucracy for not paying attention to hospital policies. Many of them find that they cannot win!

If you find a good midwife then nurture her, tell all your friends about her, tell her how good she is and above all write to the Supervisor of Midwives and tell her, too. If we are to change midwifery practice then we have to make sure they understand what it is we want.

Not all births go to plan but parents often feel positive about the outcome when they feel that they have done everything possible to give themselves a good chance. The following is a letter from Dexter who wrote:

My wife Jo was dealing with a first pregnancy, breech for seven weeks, a week overdue, and the medics are talking about automatic lithotomy, episiotomy, forceps, and induction. You told me of a GP, but he is now moving out of obstetrics and could not help us, he suggested an obstetrician, Michael, a newly arrived consultant. I phoned him and left a message, he rang me at home later and offered us an appointment that evening. He spent forty-five minutes trying to turn the baby and almost made it. He listened to our story, agreed to take us on, despite us living in another Health District outside his catchment areas, was willing to see us on the NHS, and agreed he would respect our birth plan as much as possible.

On Friday afternoon Jo's contractions began, they rumbled on, and at 9pm on Saturday we arrived at the hospital. By 4.30am on Sunday Jo had dilated from 4 to 5 centimetres, the baby's heart rate was 160–190; Jo was very tired, it being her second night without sleep. The baby was still up in the air, so we chose to have a Caesarean, although Michael was willing for the labour to continue.

Both I and Jo's sister accompanied her for the anaesthetic and the operation. I would not wish a Caesarean on anybody, but we now have a darling daughter. We learned a lot from this labour. In retrospect there are things we might have done differently, but in the circumstances we feel we did all that we reasonably could. Certainly we feel that Michael gave us the opportunity, which nobody else seemed willing to do. So, thank you for your words of encouragement and for putting us on the right trail.

WATER BIRTHS

For centuries women have been using water as a means of pain relief, in this country community midwives have used a warm bath as an alternative to drugs in labour. At the First International Home Birth Conference a woman from South America told me that, in her own home town in Guyana, it was common for the local women to go down to a particular spot on the river and give birth in the water. In view of our cooler climate, and freezing rivers, this is hardly an option in Britain! But there are alternatives.

The current enthusiasm, in this country, for water birth began when Michel Odent, an obstetrician working in a maternity unit in Pithiviers, France, observed that many women were attracted to water during their labour, some mothers used the tub purely for pain relief, while others stayed in the water to give birth to their babies.

Odent also found that when women chose to leave the water to deliver, the cooler atmosphere triggered a reflex and the baby was born almost immediately. Many women, midwives and obstetricians were worried that the baby might breathe in the water once it was born, but Odent observed that this does not happen. The baby is already in water in its mother's womb and is delivered into water of a similar temperature. The baby takes a breath when it is lifted out of the water into its mother's arms.

Arranging a water birth at home

Arranging a water birth for the birth of your baby is a relatively new experience and a growing number of parents are choosing to give birth in this manner. If you are arranging for a water birth at home you will not run into quite as many problems as some parents do when trying to arrange for this in a hospital.

There are a number of organisations which rent portable water pools, these are listed at the end of his chapter (see page 85). Individuals who have bought their own also rent out their pools and, providing you maintain a reasonable temperature, there is no reason why you should not have a water birth in your own bath, but it does make the delivery rather cramped for the midwife.

As with any home birth it is always easier to make arrangements if you have a midwife who you know is enthusiastic, but you may find that her superiors are not. In which case it is better to make the arrangements *in writing*, officials are often unwilling to put in writing statements that they have made.

The first step, therefore, will be to inform the Supervisor of Midwives, in writing, that you intend giving birth at home and that you intend having a waterbirth. The letter can be along similar lines to the letter one would write asking for a midwife for a home birth (see page 44), with an additional paragraph:

I intend having a water birth and I would appreciate it if you would allocate a midwife who has experience of, or is inter- ested in, this kind of birth.

Yours sincerely

Booking a water birth does not depend on the approval of a GP or an obstetrician, or anyone else for that matter. The decision is yours and yours alone. You may well be invited to discuss your wishes with the midwives, as delivering a baby underwater is a new experience for many of them, but their training is sufficient to deal with this kind of request. If they feel uncertain then you will be able to point out that they have a number of months to inform themselves as your baby will not be due for a while yet.

Some professionals have the idea that they have to get into the pool with the mother, this is not necessary, and there is no reason why midwives should equip themselves with a wet suit and snorkel!

If you live in Cornwall, an independent Penzance GP, Dr Roger Litchy, has for the last six years been conducting water births at home. He transports his large circular birthing pool strapped to the roof of his car, and for £750 you can hire him for pregnancy care and delivery.

There are also some independent midwives who also offer water births at home. They charge around £1,000 for pregnancy care and delivery. Further details can be found by contacting the Indepen- dent Midwives Association and the Association of Radical Midwives.

Arranging a water birth in hospital

There are some hospitals which have built their own birth pools in response to the user's demands. Hichingbrook Hospital in Hunt- ingdon was the first to do so and has had a pool since February

1987. Maidstone Hospital copied this initiative and many other hospitals have followed suit. Find out if your hospital has its own pool.

If it does not have one then all is not lost. You can bring your own, or encourage them to provide one. It is not necessary for you to book into the hospital by booking with a particular consultant obstetrician, you can book directly with the midwives. Indeed, some parents have found that the midwives were enthusiastic about a water birth but the obstetricians were not. If you decide to book with the midwives then write to the Director of Midwifery Services at the hospital concerned, and ask her to make the necessary arrangements.

If you want to book your water birth in a GP unit you do not have to get the permission of the GP or the obstetrician, despite what the staff may tell you. If, however, you have any kind of difficulty booking into a maternity unit then you should contact the Association for Improvements in the Maternity Services for help, do not battle on alone, it is very wearying and stressful.

If you find yourself arguing with the medical or midwifery staff you can bypass them and write to the Unit General Manager and seek his/her help. They are often very sympathetic.

If you do find yourself in the middle of an argument then there are two important principles by which you should act.

* ask them to state clearly what their objections are *in writing*
* ask them to produce the scientific evidence to support the criticisms they have

If you have done that and still find opposition then contact AIMS immediately. No parent should become involved in protracted arguments without support, and AIMS is the most experienced organisation around when it comes to disputes about parents' rights. At Southmead Hospital, Bristol, where they have water-birth facilities a note was stuck on the bath saying 'not to be used for delivery'. One assumes that this was an instruction to the midwives who would then ask the mother to leave the bath for delivery. What action they would take if the mother decided to stay put is anyone's guess.

In 1989 Viv contacted AIMS because she was having difficulty obtaining a water birth at home. The following is her story:

For the birth of my second baby, I thought I'd try and water birth at home. I wasn't sure if I'd want to stay in the tub for the second stage, but wanted to have the option available to me. I'd had a normal labour with my first baby (who was born in hospital), and my GP readily agreed to a home birth this time.

Antenatal care was shared between the GP practice and the community midwives (in Guy's District, SE London). Four to five months into the pregnancy I mentioned the water birth idea to the midwife I had been seeing. She was quite keen, wrote it in my notes, and I thought that was that.

Several months later, I discovered that the GP was not willing to take responsibility for a water birth and she suggested I see another, more experienced, GP in the practice. She was sympathetic, but had no experience of water births and was worried about various complications of delivery underwater. She was also worried about her legal position, should anything go wrong, and wanted to meet with the community midwife supervisor and her lawyers, to discuss all this.

Four weeks before my due date, I attended a community midwives 'tea party' (where women booked for home birth and domino get a chance to meet all the community midwives in the health district). Mrs H, the midwives' supervisor, was present and it seemed this was the first time she had heard about the water birth. She was unsure about it and said she would have to look into it further. In the meantime, my GP arranged a meeting with all the community midwives, Mrs H, Mrs H's own senior, myself and my partner. This took place just ten days before the due date. At the meeting the GP explained her reservations about the second stage in detail, but having done so, said she would attend the birth whether or not I decided to stay in the tub for delivery. The community midwives then discussed the idea of water birth amongst themselves. Some are worried about their legal position should anything go wrong in the second stage. Some were very keen on the idea and very supportive to me. Out of about fifteen midwives present, about half were doubtful or definitely unwilling to deliver a baby underwater and the other half were willing or keen to do so. None had any experience or training in water birth and this was a major concern. There was discussion of what would happen if I refused to leave the tub at the end of the first stage. Mrs H decided that at this point I should be officially asked to leave the tub, but if I decided to remain in the tub and the midwife present was unwilling to deliver the baby, she (Mrs H) would deliver the baby herself.

A few days later Mrs H agreed that only one of the midwives who was willing to deliver underwater would attend me. Mrs H herself would be present in the house, but would not come into the room unless called in.

Four days later, I went into labour. E was the community midwife on duty and was very supportive. I also had a homeopath

present, my partner and a couple of friends. I went into the tub
at about 5cm dilation and found the water very relaxing,
though not as efficient a means of pain relief as I'd hoped.
When I started feeling the urge to push and E wanted to
examine me, I decided of my own free will to get out of the
tub and stayed out for the second stage. I was not put under
any pressure at all by the midwife and soon afterwards I gave
birth, on all fours, to a healthy 8lb boy.

The midwives' anxieties about 'legal problems' were intriguing.
The following is an exchange of correspondence with the Health
Authority, in an attempt to discover precisely what 'legal problems'
there were that made the midwives so reluctant to attend; and give
some of them the opportunity to try to pressure Viv into having a
hospital birth.
    The first letter was sent to the Senior Nursing Officer at Guy's
Hospital:

I have been contacted by Mrs T who is seeking a water birth at
home, and I understand from her that you and your colleagues
are reluctant to provide the services of a midwife. I understand
from Mrs T that you perceive one of the problems as the legal
complications which might occur should there be a problem
with the birth.
    I have difficulty in understanding how a water birth would
pose legal complications for community midwives, and I would
very much appreciate it if you could explain to me just what
your anxieties about the legal issues are.

Three weeks later a reply arrived:

The midwives in Lewisham and North Southwark Health
Authority met Mrs T with her practitioner and at no time were
they reluctant to provide their services as midwives. This
meeting was amicable and constructive and my understanding
is that this is how Mrs T found the meeting.
    During this meeting the General Practitioner outlined her
legal position following advice from the Medical Defence
Union.
    I trust this clarifies the situation.

No mention has been made about the tone of the meeting and the
SNO's need to state that the meeting was 'amicable and constructive' and that was 'how Mrs T found the meeting' was a little
puzzling.

Another letter was sent:

> Thank you for your letter of 21st November describing your
> meeting with Mrs T. I did ask if you would explain just what
> the midwives' and doctor's anxieties are about the legal issues
> concerning a water birth, I note that you have not clarified this
> issue and would appreciate it if you would.

No reply was received to this request and by April 1989 the
patience was wearing a little thin. Another letter was sent:

> I first wrote to you on 31st October 1988 about your concern
> for possible legal complications which might arise should any
> problem occur during a water birth at home. In your reply of
> 21st November you did not answer my question, and I wrote
> again on 24th November asking you to explain just what these
> complications might be.
>
> On 18th January I wrote again, reminding you that I had still
> not received a reply to my query and I am now writing once
> more to ask again.
>
> As an organisation which gives women advice and help with
> childbirth issues were concerned that we have all the available
> information to hand. Clearly, if midwives feel that there are
> legal complications arising from a booked water birth at home
> we are anxious to know just what these are.
>
> I would, therefore, appreciate a reply to my letters, otherwise
> I shall be forced to conclude that these 'legal complications'
> are merely a figment of a fertile imagination and a useful
> excuse which is being used to try and dissuade women from
> booking water births.

This time the letter was copied to the Chair of the Health Authority
and the Chair of the Community Health Council.

This barb provoked, within two weeks, a reply from the Acting
Director of Midwifery Services:

> Mrs H has passed your correspondence to me in the absence of
> Miss J (the DMS) who at present is unfortunately unable to
> write to you.
>
> I would assure you that the complications that may arise are
> not a figment of a fertile imagination but more a result of
> serious thought. I would like to mention a few risks which
> would be heightened by an underwater birth:
>
> • Difficulty of ascertaining foetal distress

- Inhalation of water by the baby
- Cord around the neck of the baby
- Shoulder dystocia

- Post partum haemorrhage (difficulty in assessing true blood loss)

Having had long experience as a community midwife, I can assure you that I do believe in the efficacy of a patient laying in a warm bath during the first stage of labour and this we practised many years ago.

The Chair of the Health Authority also replied, and his reply was much more practical and forthcoming:

My I first of all offer you my sincere apologies that this matter has taken so long to reach a satisfactory resolution?

I note that you have now received a letter from Miss C, our acting Director of Midwifery Services. In her letter she outlines the main clinical potential problems which may be associated with a water birth. . . It is for these reasons that many midwives advise mothers to leave the tank for the second and third stages of labour.

There are also problems associated with the tank of water itself. These have been identified as follows:

- The weight problem. It has been estimated that a full tank of water weighs approximately one ton. Mothers wishing to book a water birth are therefore strongly advised to obtain a surveyor's report on the capacity of the floor to withstand this weight concentrated, as it would be, in one place.
- The possibility of electrocution. As you are aware, these tanks are plugged into an electricity supply in order that the water temperature is maintained. Most domestic rooms are relatively small, thus increasing the risk that splashes of water will land on electric plugs and connections with the attendant danger of electrocution.
- Risk of infection. Some tanks which are obtained on hire do not have disposable linings, and the risk of infection arising therefrom is increased. It is advisable that women seeking a water birth insist on having a disposable lining for the tank.
- It has been known for women seeking a water birth to hire a rubbish skip to be placed in a garage. Apart from the risks already outlined, a rubbish skip poses enormous problems of access and egress.

As you will readily understand, any of the problems outlined above, whether connected with clinical considerations or with the tank itself, could give rise to 'legal complications' if they contributed to harm to the baby, the mother or indeed to property. I hope that you now feel all the issues have been properly addressed, and that the advice from associations such as your own together with the advice from doctors and mid-wives will come together and result in enhanced safety and improvements in maternity care.

It is particularly helpful to have details of specific anxieties, even though they are only loosely connected with medico-legal issues. As the decision to have a water birth rests with the parents any legal complications arising from a pool cracking the ceiling, or leaking over the electrical system, would be their responsibility and nothing to do with the Health Authority.

What the midwives are worried about are complications of child-birth that could possibly arise during a water birth. Nothing to do with legal issues at all, far more to do with midwifery practice. None of the above present any legal problem whatsoever, unless, of course, a midwife was negligent in the way in which she managed any of those potential complications. A position which is no different from any other area of midwifery practice.

It is a pity that some midwife managers (and practising mid-wives) confuse legal issues with midwifery practice, and use the threat of potential legal action as a bludgeon to persuade mothers to give up and go into hospital like good little girls.

It is not necessary to spend money hiring a water pool. It is perfectly possible to have a water birth in your own bath at home, a practice that was not unknown in this country long before Odent drew attention to it. If, however, you do decide to hire your own pool there are four main centres for pool hire. They also give help and advice to parents who are having difficulties booking a water birth:

The Active Birth Centre. 55 Dartmouth Park Road, London NW5 ISL, 071-267-3006. Pools can be hired for £125, plus £20 for a disposable plastic liner. It is reserved for four weeks, a fortnight either side of the due date. They also sell pools.

Birthworks. Hill House, Folleigh Lane, Long Ashton, Bristol BS18 9JB, 0272-394202. Two types of tub are available, a circular one and a rectangular one designed for hospitals. The charge is £35 a week.

Splashdown Birth Pool Hire. 17 Wellington Terrace, Harrow on the

Hill, HA1 3EP, 081-422-9308. The pools are specially designed for labour and birth by Keith Brainin of the Active Birth Centre in association with Michel Odent. The pools come with a sterilised disposable inner liner, and they will deliver a pool anywhere.

The Birthing Tub Company. Pakyns Lodge, Albourne Road, Hurst-pierpoint, West Sussex BN6 9ET, 0273-835245. They charge £100 plus a delivery charge.

Pools which use recirculating water systems are difficult to keep clean, and a number of hospitals have been wary of using them. Research evidence has shown that recirculating water pumps do present problems, but so far, it is a theoretical one. We know of no woman or baby, to date, who has caught an infection from a water pool. We do know of many women and babies, who have not had water births, but who leave hospital with hospital-borne infections.

10

MEDICAL RESEARCH

Since the 1950s the development of obstetric technology has blossomed. Many of the new technologies have been developed to assist women and babies who have had problems during pregnancy or childbirth. Unfortunately, the desire to help the minority has spilled over to such an extent that a new technology is often rushed into general use long before it has been properly evaluated – the misuse of ultrasound and foetal monitoring are but two classic examples.

Medical research is not a benign activity where new technology and new procedures are carefully evaluted and, when a conclusion is reached, steps taken to ensure that the new development is appropriately used. Instead poorly controlled trials take place throughout the country in most hospitals all of the time, depending upon the whims of the staff involved and often the enthusiasm of the drug or medical equipment manufacturers who are keen to support trials of their products.

The take-up of new technology and new procedures, therefore, depends very much on fashion, publicity and medical equipment manufacturers. In other words, the sooner everyone knows about a new development the sooner the manufacturers can produce and market it and the sooner women will be asking for it. The easier it will be to claim the 'we cannot carry out a randomised controlled trial to evaluate the benefits and risks properly because it is now in general use and it will be unethical to do so'. The ethics of widely using an unevaluated technique on women and babies are not considered; such an approach condones the use of women and babies as guinea pigs in unscientific medical experimentation. The damage this approach has caused to hundreds and thousands of women and babies in Britain has still not been properly assessed.

Medical trials take place throughout the country in most most hospitals, most of the time, although it must be said that obstetricians are the least likely of all medical specialists to conduct randomised controlled trials to evaluate their practice. It is usual for any doctor wishing to undertake a particular piece of research to approach his/her local medical ethics committee and seek approval. Having obtained approval the doctor can then go ahead with his/her trial. S/he does not, necessarily, have to obtain your consent to take part in a trial but in most cases informed consent would be obtained. There have also been examples of medical trials being conducted without ethics committee approval.

THE ISSUES

Obstetric care is an area of medicine in which enormous numbers of procedures have been introduced without proper evaluation. This has resulted in thousands of women and babies being subjected to technologies that are often of questionable value and sometimes cause considerable risk to particular individuals.

The Committee on Safety of Medicines was established to control the use and introduction of drugs in medical practice; it issues licences for new drugs and goes some way towards controlling the development and marketing, although many would argue not nearly far enough. Where medical technology is concerned, however, there is no parallel body and no one to control the introduction of new technologies and procedures. For too long the medical profession and the medical manufacturers have been allowed carte blanche to introduce whatever wonderful new, unevaluated, technological development they like. It is time that a committee was established for the evaluation of medical technologies. That way the proliferation of unevaluated new machines could be controlled and the users could look forward to the day when no new machine would be introduced into general use without first having been subjected to a randomised controlled trial to establish its worth. Such a committee could prevent future generations of women and babies being used as guinea pigs in uncontrolled medical experimentation.

At the moment, much of the medical research carried out is determined mainly by men, the majority of whom are doctors and members of pharmaceutical firms, machine manufacturers and other commercial interests. It is hardly surprising, therefore, that little attention is paid to the kind of research the users would like to see. For instance, there are very few good studies on diets of pregnant women, on the problems of morning sickness and the effects of disturbing women during labour by a continuous stream of strange faces. Thankfully there are some members of the medical and midwifery professions who are concerned about addressing the kinds of studies the users want and are interested in the question of properly informing the public about the nature of medical research.

YOUR RIGHTS

Having been given information (usually verbal) about the trial, you have the right to refuse to take part. If you decide to take part in the trial then, at a later date, decide to withdraw you have an absolute right so to do.

Carrying out research and giving treatment to any individual without consent, and in a child's case the assent of the parents or guardian, leaves a Health Authority open to a charge of assault.

RANDOMISED CONTROLLED TRIALS

New technologies and new procedures are being introduced all the time and they have to be evaluated, preferably before their wide-spread acceptance. In order to do that properly the procedures have to be tried out on people, otherwise there is no way of telling whether or not they are effective.

Over the years the medical profession has developed a technique called a randomised controlled trial. This technique usually involves randomly allocating people to two groups: a control group (usually a group which will have a standard treatment in current use) and the research group which will have the new treatment. Calculations are made about the number of people needed to show whether the new treatment is effective, and once that number is reached it is possible to tell whether the new treatment works. Sometimes it is possible to find that out well before the end of the trial and some trials have stopped before reaching their planned number.

Such planning for medical trials usually takes place within the confines of the medical establishment an it is unusual for any user group to be approached in these early stages.

The chorionic villus sampling trial, which started in 1986, was a very unusual and important example of the medical profession approaching user groups for help and advice during the planning stages.

Chorionic villus sampling is a technique by which the obstetrician is able to take a small amount of developing cells (chorionic villus) and examine them to determine whether the mother is carrying a baby with a genetic defect. The test is done when the woman is about ten weeks pregnant (see page 23 for further details).

The trial organisers drafted an information leaflet to be given to every woman who took part in the trial and the user groups were able to comment on the leaflet and make suggestions and amendments.

It should be a principle of all good scientific research that everyone approached to take part in a clinical trial should be given an information leaflet telling them as much as possible about the trial, so that they can consider whether they wish to take part. Leaflets also enable user groups can check on the kind of information that women are receiving. When verbal consent is sought and the information is given verbally it is very difficult to check what trial recruits have been told; some researchers in their enthusiasm to recruit people to their trial are not always as forthcoming about the disadvantages as they might be.

Although it is not always possible to give written information for all studies and trials, it is certainly possible for the majority.

Uncontrolled trials

Uncontrolled trials are trials where the staff feel they ought to try out a procedure on a number of women and babies to see how it goes; no attempt is made to compare the outcome with a comparable group; and very little information is given to those who are asked to take part in the trial.

If people involved in controlled trials are to receive leaflets telling them about the trial, then surely people involved in uncontrolled trials should also receive information leaflets. The following has been suggested:

> Doctors at this and every hospital will come to a decision about what type(s) of care to offer you in a variety of ways. Sometimes there will be good evidence of the effectiveness and relative safety of the treatment recommended; more often, doctors will be influenced by tradition, prejudice, fashion or bad evidence in making their recommendations; occasionally doctors who want to ensure that they maximise the chances of your having whichever turns out to be the best of alternative treatments will select your treatment at random from the likely best alternatives. If you want to know anything about the basis upon which your treatment has been selected; or about the alternatives and their relative merits and disadvantages; or what doctors here are doing to try to minimise their unintended mistakes and protect their patients from them, then do not hesitate to ask for this information.

At the moment, the only people interested in giving out information leaflets are those people who are currently involved in controlled trials. There has yet to be formulated a means of dealing with those who are happily conducting uncontrolled trials, and by so doing are using pregnant women and babies as guinea pigs in uncontrolled experimentation.

Consenting to trials

If you are approached and asked to take part in a study or trial, controlled or uncontrolled, you should ask the following questions before deciding:

- has this study been approved by the Ethics Committee?
- what written information do they have about the study?
- what are the known risks, to you and/or your baby, of having the new treatment?
- what are the known risks, to you and/or your baby, of having the established treatment?
- what are the hoped for benefits, for you and/or your baby, of the new treatment?
- what are the hoped for benefits, for you and/or your baby, of the established treatment?
- will you have time to go away and think about your decision and consult with other people before deciding whether or not to take part?

If the trial has not been approved by the Ethics Committee then you should enquire why not. As a general rule all trials should be submitted for the Ethics Committee's approval and you should be wary of any that have not. CERES, a user group concerned about ethics in medical research should be informed. Their address is PO Box 1365, London N16 OBW, 0732-458021.

It is important that anyone asked to take part in a trial is given written information about the purposes of the trial and the potential risks and benefits to those who are being recruited to take part. No matter how fair a doctor or researcher tries to be, they are unlikely to be able to present you with a balanced argument upon which you can make a decision; it will tend to be coloured by what they want you to do, no matter how hard they try to be neutral. This is why written information is important, it gives you the opportunity of seeing a balanced statement and also you have the chance of going away and thinking about it before making up your mind.

Once you have had answers to the above questions, preferably in writing, then you will be in a better position to decide whether or not you wish to take part in the study/trial.

There are, however, many medical trials taking place in hospitals all over the country at this moment, for which no information leaflets are produced and consent is obtained verbally. There are even controlled and uncontrolled trials taking place (particularly in intensive and special care baby units) of which parents are completely unaware. They have never been approached for assent to the treatment.

Continuing discussions are taking place about the best approach in informing the users about medical studies/trials. The Association for Improvements in the Maternity Services has suggested that every hospital in Britain should display a notice in the antenatal clinics stating that at this moment the hospital is currently conducting a trial on . . . and anyone wanting information can apply to . . . This action will at least ensure that women begin to understand that there are studies and trials taking place and will give them opportunity to think about the question before they are approached to take part.

11
COMMON OBSTETRIC PROCEDURES AND TECHNOLOGIES

> The male practitioner, adding insult to injury, was so adept at concealing his errors with a 'cloud of hard words and scientific jargon', that the injured patient herself was convinced that she could not thank him enough for the mischief he had done (Elizabeth Nihill, Midwife, Hotel Dieu, Paris, 1761).

Many people choose to have their babies in hospital because they believe it is safer. Obstetricians over the years have constantly threatened women with death and disaster if they risk anything other than obstetric care. In reality, hospitals carry their own risks, not only of hospital bred infections (many of which do not exist outside hospitals) but also of letting the patient in for treatments which are often unnecessary, inappropriate and until very recently largely unevaluated.

Obstetric technology was developed to help those women and babies who had problems. Unfortunately, it is then often used on just about everyone, on the principle that if it is good in one instance it must be better in all! At that point, the risks of technology begin to exceed the risks of the condition it was designed to prevent.

It is always difficult for the individual mother to determine whether or not a procedure is being used as a routine because the standard response from most staff to any questions is 'we only use it when indicated, never as a routine'. Yet, if you obtain a copy of the hospital statistics you will find that in many hospitals the view of 'necessary' is very high.

As a rule of thumb, any procedure carried out on more than 20 per cent of women and babies is an over-used procedure: you should think very hard about what you can do to ensure that any procedure offered you is only done when absolutely necessary.

Some questions you can ask are, why *in my case* is this procedure considered necessary? What are the indications that my baby is distressed and this procedure is needed? What scientific evidence do you have to support your proposal?

It is not the purpose of this handbook to go into great detail about the pros and cons of each procedure. The very best books you can read on the subject of the risks and benefits of obstetric technology are *Birthrights* (1989) and *A Guide to Effective Care in Pregnancy and Childbirth* (1989). In *Birthrights* Sally Inch describes very well how women by agreeing to one intervention often find themselves on the slippery slope of *needing* more interventions. Her book discusses, at length, the advantages and disadvantages of obstetric technology and modern management of labour. The second book, *A Guide to Effective Care in Pregnancy and Childbirth*, by three eminent doctors, Enkin, Keirse and Chalmers, provides a scientific analysis of the studies which have been done in maternity care, and draws conclusions about their effectiveness and use in current obstetric practice. If you have been prescribed a form of treatment and you are doubtful about its value this is the book to consult.

The following are some of the more common procedures and technologies and some brief information about them:

AMNIOTOMY (BREAKING THE WATERS)

Artifical early rupture of the membranes, as a routine process, is not scientifically justified (World Health Organisation, 1985).

Breaking the waters is one of the common routine procedures carried out in many British hospitals and women are unaware of the way in which it can pervert the course of a normal labour. Professor Roberto Caldeyro-Barcia (the past president of the International Confederation of Obstetricians and Gynaecologists) in a paper about the adverse effects of amniotomy stated that

Amniotomy is still being systematically executed despite several publications demonstrating that it disturbs the normal balance of pressure received by the uterine contents (foetus, placenta and cord) during uterine contractions and bearing-down efforts, thus facilitating the uneven compression and deformation of the foetal head, and the occlusion (compression) of umbilical vessels.'

Enkin, Keirse and Chalmers in *A Guide to Effective Care in Pregnancy and Childbirth* state

> The main disadvantage of amniotomy when used alone for the induction of labour is the unpredictable, and occasionally long, interval to the onset of labour-like uterine activity, and thus to delivery.

Amniotomy is more likely to be used in conjunction with oxytocin for the induction or acceleration of labour (see page 114, Induction and Acceleration).

There may be an occasion later in the labour when breaking the waters will assist you. You have the right to ask the staff why they are recommending breaking the waters and what evidence they have to justify their proposed action.

If you are not satisfied that they are recommending the procedure in the best interests of you or your baby you have the right to refuse.

BREECH BIRTHS

Twenty years ago midwives delivered breech babies of multiparous women at home as a normal procedure. Since then the majority of women have been booked into hospital for childbirth and the obstetricians decided that breech would now be considered an abnormal delivery. It became an obstetric issue, and in some hospitals all breech babies are automatically scheduled to be delivered by Caesarean section. There is no scientific evidence to justify this policy.

In the 1960s and 1970s it was common for women to be confined to bed for their labour, flat on their backs, and when the baby was near delivery the women's feet would be put in stirrups. This meant that the woman was essentially pushing the baby uphill and, because she was flat on her back, the pelvic diameter was reduced. For the breech baby this practice created a number of serious difficulties and increased the risks. The obstetricians sought to solve the problems they had created by the increased use of forceps and Caesarean sections.

If you are expecting a baby, and it is in the breech position by 36 weeks, there are a number of ways of encouraging it to turn. Janet Balaskas and Yehudi Gordon in their book *The Encyclopedia of Pregnancy and Birth* describe an alternative method. Lie on your back with a pillow under your head and bottom. Gently massage your belly in the direction in which you want the baby to move. Your midwife will be able to tell you which way the baby is lying.

Once the baby has turned, stop the exercise and squat to encourage the head to engage.

Acupuncturists recommend the application of pressure, heat or acupuncture needles to a point on the outer edge of the little toe to encourage a breech baby to turn. This can be done in combination with the above exercise.

Effective Care in Pregnancy and Childbirth describes how traditional midwives in Gazankulu, South Africa, attempt to correct breech presentations during labour by manually shaking the uterus while the mother is in the knee-elbow position on the floor.

If you are told that you are expecting a breech baby and you are not happy about the proposed care you can ask for a second opinion. It is better to seek a second opinion from an obstetrician at a different hospital; when they work together in the same place they are not so likely to challenge their colleague's care. Before you book the second opinion check *his/her* Caesarean section rates first.

When assessing the potential for a normal vaginal delivery the obstetrician and midwives will be considering the following:

- The size of the baby, if it is too big or too small, i.e. over 8lb 13oz (4kg) or under 4lb 6oz (2kg).
- Your baby is not premature, i.e. less than 37 weeks.
- The size of your pelvis is adequate.
- Your pregnancy has proceeded normally.
- The baby does not have an abnormality which is causing the breech presentation – a *very* rare occurrence.

Having checked that there are no problems, other than the obstetric management of a breech birth, you can ask for a midwife delivery; cancel your booking with the consultant and book directly with the midwives. You can write to the Director of Midwifery Services at the hospital along the following lines:

Dear

I am expecting a breech baby on . . . . . . and have been booked for delivery with Mr/s . . . . I do not feel that the care offered, electronic foetal monitoring throughout labour, forceps delivery/Caesarean section (include whichever is applicable) is appropriate in my case.

I would prefer my baby to be delivered vaginally, by a midwife, and I would appreciate it if you would allocate to me a midwife who has experience of a vaginal breech delivery.

Should any complication arise during the labour or birth

which would necessitate consultant involvement I would be willing, in those circumstances, for him/her to attend.

Your sincerely

Women who have active births greatly increase their chances of a vaginal delivery and reduce the risks of complication. If you have decided to choose to have a vaginal birth you can also check that your midwife has read *Community Midwifery* by Mary Cronk and Caroline Flint, this book has an excellent section on how to deliver a breech vaginally.

BIRTH POSITIONS

There is only one position worse than lying a woman flat on her back for delivery and that is hanging her by her heels from a chandelier (Professor Roberto Caldeyro Barcia, past President of the International Confederation of Obstetricians and Gynaecologists).
Pregnant women should not be put in a lithotomy position (flat on their backs) during labour or delivery. They should be encouraged to walk about during labour and each woman must freely decide which position to adopt during delivery (World Health Organisation, 1985).

The blame for the current obstetric fashion for lying a woman on her back for labour and delivery can be laid at the door of King Louis XIV of France. He wanted to watch his mistresses' babies delivered, but as he had to peep through a curtain (because men were not allowed into the delivery room) he could not see very much. So he ordered that the women deliver lying on the bed. The suggestion soon became a fashion and, of course, it offered the obstetrician considerable advantages (an immobile woman, and an uninterrupted view of the perineum).
It is only in the last 10 years or so that women have been vociferously challenging the assertion that all women should give birth in a bed and immobile. Michel Odent, a French surgeon, reminded us that a vertical position is much more favourable for childbirth (although many midwives are concerned about attending a woman whose perineum they cannot see easily). Janet Balaskas has pioneered and promoted the idea of an 'Active Birth', her book *The New Active Birth* describes very well how women can assist labour and benefit considerably by staying active and mobile during labour and delivery.

In order to demonstrate how progressive and responsive they are to women's needs, many hospitals soon introduced a birthing chair. Birthing chairs or stools have a long history and were used extensively in the middle ages. It is possible to buy a birthing stool for about £36: it looks like a kidney shaped coffee table (indeed, many women use them as coffee tables afterwards). However, the hospitals decided to respond to the enthusiastic inventions of the medical equipment companies. The result was 'Borning Beds' (£6,950) and a variety of horrifying chairs designed to 'help' labouring woman.

Naturally, the obstetric birthing chairs were incredibly expensive and unevaluated. After a time, some hospitals carried out evaluations and discovered that in some of the chairs the women suffered more tears. Surprise, surprise! If you are sitting in a chair in which your legs are held apart in a fixed position, you must be putting quite a strain on the perineal muscles. The point about the birthing stool is that the woman is free to move about as she wishes. With an obstetric birthing chair women are fixed into a position a couple of feet off the ground (and guess who has his/her finger on the control button?).

Some hospitals also decided that they could not allow student midwives to use the birthing stool until a protocol had been devised. So much for allowing the woman to be free to do what she wants! Sadly, in some hospitals the birthing stools are gathering dust in cupboards. Many midwives hate using them and you have to search about to find out if the hospital has one. If it is in use when you go into labour, that is your bad luck.

You could, of course, buy one yourself and take it with you; alternatively, you could take in a bean bag. Many women find bean bags very useful. You can push the bed into a corner and sit on the bean bag on the floor. You are then in the enviable position of doing what you wish, and if you decided that you do want to go and lie down on the bed then you have that option too.

Comparison of conventional versus alternative (squatting) deiivery management (Haddad, 1985):

	Conventionally managed women	Alternatively managed women
Cervical dilatation on admission to labour ward	Lesser	Greater
Number having labour induced	Higher	Lower

Meconium-stained liquor	More common	Less common
Use of electronic foetal monitoring	More common	Less common
Use of oxytocin to induce or augment	Significantly higher	Significantly lower
Detection of foetal heart rate abnormalities	More common	Less common
Use of analgesia	Significantly more	Significantly less
Number of achieving spontaneous vaginal delivery	Significantly lower	Significantly higher
Apgar score at 1, 3, and 5 min (independently assessed)	Significantly Lower	Significantly Higher

CAESAREAN SECTIONS

The first recorded Caesarean section, in which both mother and baby survived, was carried out by Mary Dunally, an Irish midwife, in 1738. It was an operation which was carried out as a last desperate measure to save the child, and usually only after the mother had died.

Over two hundred years later the introduction of improved anaesthetics meant that the risk of Caesarean section was considerably reduced. Although, the overall rate of maternal death associated with Caesarean delivery has changed little during the last twenty years.

During the early 1950s the Caesarean section rate was 2.2 per cent, but by 1983 the rates within England had climbed to a range from 8.6 per cent to 11.5 per cent. In Scotland the rates varied between 8.7 per cent and 17.4 per cent. The rate amongst women giving birth in pay beds in NHS hospitals was 19.6 per cent, compared with 9 per cent for ordinary NHS patients. The Maternity Alliance's report *Changing Childbirth* – Interventions in Labour in England and Wales shows that Caesarean sections in consultant units range from 0 per cent to a staggering 25 per cent in one particular hospital.

It has been claimed that Caesarean sections have contributed to the reduction in infant mortality rates, yet there is no scientific evidence to support this, and the wide variation in Caesarean rates reflects the considerable differences in obstetric practice around the country.

One of the reasons for the increase in Caesareans is the fashion for induction and acceleration of labour, particularly for 'overdue' babies. Mr John Studd, consultant obstetrician at King's College Hospital, said 'it is a disaster to induce routinely overdue babies. I am very much opposed to it, because it produces prolonged labour and foetal distress'. In a study of 2,000 women 142 went to 42 weeks, 46 were induced, the rest delivered spontaneously, all before 44 weeks. He found that the group which was not induced had shorter labours and there were fewer Caesareans.

A proportion of the increase in Caesarean sections is accounted for by the increasing tendency to deliver twins, breech babies, and very low birthweight babies by Caesarean, and a policy of 'once a Caesarean always a Caesarean'. There is considerable dispute within the medical profession about the values of these policies. Any woman facing such action should ask for a second opinion.

Results from randomised controlled trials of electronic foetal monitoring have shown an association between raised Caesarean rates and the use of continuous electronic foetal monitoring.

Dr Robert Atlay, a former honorary secretary of the Royal College of Obstetricians and Gynaecologists, commenting on a Radio 4 programme, said 'The high Caesar rate is due to lack of training of young doctors in dealing with difficult deliveries.' Some obstetricians have identified staff shortages, in which junior staff are left in charge and are, therefore, more likely to carry out a Caesarean than bide their time or carry out a ventouse delivery. Part of this problem has been identified as lack of consultant obstetricians on the labour wards and leaving the work to the junior staff. An increasing problem since the relaxation of NHS consultants' private practice conditions in 1980.

One of the most common reasons given for the increase in Caesarean sections is fear of litigation. A claim which followed the judgement in 1978 in the case of Jordan v. Whitehouse. The case was brought following an attempted vaginal delivery with forceps. The baby was born brain damaged. The parents initially won their case but it was overturned on appeal. Nevertheless, some obstetricians felt sufficiently threatened that they became reluctant to undertake difficult forceps deliveries.

According to Doris Haire, President of the American Foundation for Maternal and Child Health, similar claims are made in America where obstetricians frequently contend that the high rate of Caesarean section in the US is an attempt to forestall medical malpractice suits. They tend to ignore the fact that in the US there has been only a 1 per cent per capita rise in medical malpractice suits filed against doctors over the past ten years. They also ignore the fact that in Canada the rate of Caesarean section is almost identical to that in the US, despite Canada having a legal system which makes it prohibitively expensive for an injured patient to file a malpractice suit against a negligent doctor.

Although maternal death following Caesarean section is rare it is, none the less, more dangerous for the mother than having a vaginal delivery, and for some there are problems of wound inflammation (17.4 per cent) minor sepsis (5.1 per cent) and major sepsis (1 per cent).

Caesarean sections represent the pinnacle of interventionist obstetric care, and the costs, to the National Health Service, of this epidemic of Caesareans is enormous. Dr Iain Chalmers, Director of the National Perinatal Epidemiology Unit, has estimated that

> if, in 1976, obstetricians in England and Wales had performed Caesarean operations at the same rate as their American colleagues, an additional 35,000 women would have been subjected to this major surgical procedure at an additional cost to the health services of about £18 million.

The current rate of Caesarean operations is 62,000 a year.

For the families there is the additional expense of visiting the mother in hospital, care for the other children while she is there, time off work for the partner, additional care in the home, and because many women fail to breastfeed, the additional expense of buying formula food.

There was a time when Caesarean sections were presented as the 'Rolls Royce of maternity care.' In Brazil women are exhorted to have Caesareans so that they can keep their vaginas 'honeymoon fresh'. Fortunately, British women have not been subjected to such 'hype'. Caesarean sections are traumatic experiences, which leave many women with considerable hurdles to overcome, at the very time she should be at the peak of health. Having suffered major surgery the mother is expected to be on her feet as soon as possible, finding that she has taken on a 24-hour demanding new job. A job at which she is expected to succeed with little or no additional assistance. It is hardly surprising, therefore, that researchers have found higher levels of post-natal depression amongst women who have had Caesareans, fewer mothers continuing breastfeeding, and many experiencing greater difficulties in relating to their babies.

In order to try and stop this epidemic of Caesarean it has been suggested that there should be a greater use of randomised controlled trials, to assess the value of some of the routines used in British hospitals, together with local and national audit of operation rates. However, one of the greatest effects on practice, in the past, has been achieved by user demand. There is a great deal that you can do to avoid an emergency Caesarean section.

What is an avoidable Caesarean section?

Very little public attention has been focused on avoidable Caesarean sections. Apart from the planned ones, the majority of Caesarean sections are carried out as an emergency to save the baby. However, low-risk, fit and healthy women in consultant units or teaching hospitals often find themselves subjected to the vast range of largely unevaluated routine procedures. There will be a proportion of them who will find the labour going disasterously wrong and having to be rescued, by having a Caesarean section, from the crisis the procedures have provoked. These are the avoidable Caesarean sections.

A study by Barrett *et al* (Vol. 336, 1990), published in *The Lancet*, showed that one in three Caesarean sections is unnecessary. Just as disturbing was the analysis of the auditors' decisions. When faced with identical information at a different time the auditors, themselves, were inconsistent in a quarter of their findings.

How to reduce the risk of having to have an emergency Caesarean section

* Find out what the Caesarean section rates are in your local hospital. Consultant units and teaching hospitals have the highest Caesarean section rates of all, ranging from 0 per cent to 25 per cent. The lowest Caesarean section rates can be found amongst low-risk women who book into general practitioner units, but these units are being closed down as fast as the Health authorities can manage it, so that they can force all women into their high-risk, centralised obstetric and teaching hospitals.

* If you really have no choice but to go into the local consultant unit which has a high rate of Caesarean sections (i.e. over 10 per cent) find out what the rates are by consultant. Consultant obstetricians' practice varies considerably, and within any unit there is usually at least one particular consultant who is less interventionist than his/her colleagues. You can then ask to be booked with him/her.

* If all the consultants have little to choose between them, write to the Director of Midwifery Services and book directly under midwifery care. You do not need to book under the care of a consultant obstetrician, and if the unit is trying to improve the quality of its care then it will be introducing midwifery teams, so that low-risk women can have continuity of midwifery care. If they do not have such a scheme you have now given them the opportunity of introducing one.

- Have your baby at home or in a GP unit.
- If you have to book into a consultant unit or teaching hospital book a domino delivery or book for midwifery care only.
- Read Janet Balaskas's book *Active Birth*, Sally Inch's book *Birth-rights* and Marjorie Tew's book *Safer Childbirth*? Between these books and the one you are now reading you should acquire a good understanding of the issues and what you can do about it.

Conscious during a Ceasarean section

In October 1981 AIMS received a letter from a Mrs McCobb who had written to a magazine *Maternity and Mothercraft* about being conscious during a Caesarean section under a general anaesthetic. They had advised her to contact AIMS. No one in AIMS had ever heard of anyone who had had this experience before, but Mrs McCobb told us that she knew of another woman who had a similar experience a week previously. She was advised to find the woman and it took her nine weeks to do so. Although she knew the woman's name she did not know where she lived but a letter in the local paper resulted in Mrs Ackers making contact.

It was clear that if there were two mothers who were conscious during a general anaesthetic there might be more. A carefully worded letter was placed in the local press asking any other mothers who had had similar experiences to make contact. Within a few weeks fourteen other women made contact. Twelve of the women had had Caesarean sections, two had had sterilisations.

The experiences of the women varied a great deal. One wrote to say that, although she had been conscious, she had already lost three children (this baby survived) and she felt grateful to the doctors; she described the experience as 'unpleasant'.

The experiences of women who have been conscious during a Caesarean section under a general anaesthetic range from those who woke up for a short period, were aware of what was happening but were in no pain; those who woke up for a short period, experienced a little pain to a great deal of pain, and the very rare instances of those women who were conscious all the way through their Caesarean sections and who were also in considerable pain. The drugs used for general anaesthetic cause a loss of conscious-ness and paralysis. In these cases there had been an insufficient dose to cause complete loss of consciousness but the paralysing drug was very effective, the women were unable to alert the doctors. An alert anaesthetist will, however, be suspicious when the woman's blood pressure increases.

Other women described their experiences, although they were not as traumatic as Mrs Acker's, only one was conscious throughout the operation, the others were conscious for varying periods of time.

Some of the women said that they were pleased to discover that they were not alone in their experiences, not because they wished such a ghastly experience upon anyone else, but because, having been told by just about everyone that they imagined it, they finally had confirmation that what they had experienced really did happen. It was a considerable relief to realise that they were not going mad. Three of the women were having psychiatric treatment, one for a phobia about death. Three other women specifically mentioned that they were suffering from nightmares and two of them are terrified of hospitals and operations. One of the women has been sterilised because she could not bear the thought of any subsequent children; indeed, three of the mothers stated that they could not face the thought of having any more children, and a few mentioned that their sex lives had been seriously affected.

By June 1985 Mrs Acker's case came to court. She described how she felt the first incision, how she wanted to scream but could not; how she felt them lift the baby out and felt every one of the stitches when they were sewing her up. The operation lasted 75 minutes and during that time she lay in agony, unable to alert the attendants. In describing her state of consciousness a consultant anaesthetist, Professor Robinson said: 'She was not just aware, she was fully conscious.' Mrs Ackers stated, 'The pain was terrible. It seemed to go on for ages.' The judge, Mr Justice Russell, was horrified and said, 'What should have been a joyous occasion turned out to be a terrifying, agonising experience.' He awarded her £13,775 damages. The Health Authority had admitted liability (although in the early stages of the action they had offered £1,500 as an out-of-court settlement, they then paid into court £6,000 and eventually increased their offer to £10,000 on the steps of the court).

Following the High Court judgement the news media, which had not been remotely interested in this case *before* the High Court settlement, went wild. The case was reported in the national newspapers and on radio and TV. It prompted other women to contact AIMS. Altogether seventy-three women made contact, as well as a number who contacted the solicitor directly. It was felt that it would be helpful to them to get together and discuss their experiences. AIMS arranged a meeting in Manchester with the solicitor who dealt with the legal action, Ann Alexander, the consultant anaesthetist, Professor Robinson, and a sympathetic psychiatrist, Dr Downham who had been helping some of the women.

The meeting was an enormous success, many of the women were relieved to be able to discuss their own experiences with others, and be reassured that what they had suffered during the operation and subsequently was not unusual. They discovered that one of the common reactions from the profession was 'You must have been dreaming' or 'it could not possibly happen', or they simply changed the subject.

As a result of this case the medical profession has acknowledged that awareness under a general anaesthetic can occur in around 5 per cent of cases. The midwifery profession is now far more sympathetic and supportive of women who tell them that they were conscious, and encourage them to talk about it at the time.

It was clear from listening to the experiences of these mothers that it is very unhelpful, and very damaging, to suggest that the mother was lying or dreaming. Some doctors have made comments suggesting that making these experiences public would encourage 'copy-cat' cases. In all the contact AIMS has had with women who have said they have had this experience not one has been lying. In every case the woman has been able to give details of their experiences which no ordinary woman would have known about, unless she has been in the operating theatre and awake.

The likelihood of this kind of experience happening to you is extremely remote, but there is, apart from the usual childbirth groups which can help, a specific group of women who are giving help and support. It is called The Wide Awake Club, 22 King's Lea, Heath Charnock, Adlington, Lancs, PR7 4EH.

Vaginal birth after Caesarean section (VBAC)

The accepted obstetric view 'once a Caesarean always a Caesarean' is being challenged by increasing numbers of pregnant women, as well as professionals. The major anxiety is that of scar rupture. Yet, *Effective Care in Pregnancy and Childbirth* states,

> To put these rates into perspective, the probability of requiring an emergency Caesarean section for other acute conditions (foetal distress, cord prolapse, or antepartum haemorrhage) in any women giving birth, is approximately 2.7 per cent, or 30 times as high as the risk of uterine rupture with a trial of labour.

Women who have had more than one Caesarean section often express doubt that a VBAC can be achieved in their case. A report in the American *Journal of Obstetrics and Gynaecology* showed that for women who had had two or more previous Caesarean sections 77 per cent achieved a VBAC.

A number of lay groups have been formed to support women

who want a VBAC, one of the most active, the Caesarean Support Network, is conducting a survey of hospitals asking them what their policies are. The replies they received have been quite depressing. The most common response appears to be:

- you will have an intravenous drip inserted into your vein for the administration of glucose and water, drugs, etc.
- You will have continuous electronic foetal monitoring, including a foetal scalp electrode.
- The membranes will probably be ruptured if they have not already done so.
- You will be starved, but allowed sips of water.

Research evidence shows that each one of the above interventions can pervert the course of a normal labour and *increase* the likelihood of needing a Caesarean section.

There are many who feel that a VBAC is best achieved by encouraging the mother to have an active birth. The above interventions should be restricted to occasions where there are clear indications that they are really needed.

The Encyclopaedia of Pregnancy and Birth states,

Using upright positions in such a labour is not only safe but preferable. An active birth will usually shorten labour, help the uterus work better and relieve pressure on the scar. In the second stage, an upright supported squat is ideal. If there are any difficulties the doctor may then consider using ventous to help reduce the strain and help the delivery.

If you want a VBAC for your next delivery ask your local hospital for a description of the routine care they would give you. If it includes any of the above list you can ask them for the scientific evidence which supports their proposals. If they are not supportive of what you want you can approach another hospital. Also contact the Caesarean Support Network or the VBAC Contact Group or other user groups which can give advice and help. The more information you have the better. There are a number of excellent books about VBAC.

All women wanting a VBAC face the possibility that they may not succeed. It is, therefore, important not to arrange a VBAC with unrealistic expectations and become overconfident. While confidence is important, it can be devastating and deeply disappointing when one does not get what one wants. For some women a vaginal birth may be only a slight possibility, but they often feel better and positive about having to have another Caesarean section when they have been well informed, well prepared and involved in the decisions which were made during labour and have discussed and consulted with other supportive people.

ELECTRONIC FOETAL MONITORING

> In the light of the evidence now available it is our view that there can be little justification for the use of continuous electronic foetal heart-rate monitoring without the facilities to assess foetal acid-base status (foetal blood sampling) when a foetus is thought to be compromised (Dermot Macdonald *et al.*, 1983).

> Continuous electronic foetal monitoring is not a panacea but it does have advantages. The level of staffing in many labour wards in this country is abysmally low. Therefore we need electronic monitoring (Professor Stuart Campbell, Kings College Hospital, *Guardian*, 2nd March 1990).

An electronic foetal monitor consists of two small devices which are strapped to the mother's abdomen with broad belts; one will record the contractions and the other will record simultaneously the baby's heart rate. If they are working properly. These devices are connected by thin leads to the monitoring machine which will be at the bedside. This will print out a continuous recording of the contractions and heart rate on graph paper. An internal foetal scalp electrode can also be used. This will attach an electrode on to whichever part of the baby is presenting and a lead will attach it to the monitor, which, if it is working properly, will record the baby's heart rate.

Over the last twenty years electronic foetal monitoring has become a standard piece of labour-ward equipment and many obstetricians have never worked without them. Midwives have been deskilled in the use of Pinard stethoscopes and they too have become reliant on this only recently evaluated technology. It is another example of a technology which was introduced and widely used without a proper evaluation. In 1983, however, the results of a large randomised controlled trial of intrapartum electronic foetal heart rate monitoring (EFM) were published (Macdonald, 1983). It was found that

- Mothers allocated to EFM were significantly less likely to receive pethidine for analgesia and had significantly shorter labours, but were significantly more likely to be delivered by forceps, and slightly more likely to be delivered by Caesarean section (hence the shorter labours).
- There were significantly fewer neonatal convulsions among those

allocated to EFM but there were more deaths ascribed to trauma in this group.

• Routine EFM with foetal blood sampling reduced the frequency of neonatal convulsions by 56 per cent (in the study a total of 39 babies suffered from convulsions and 12,960 women took part). It was estimated that in order to prevent one case of neonatal convulsions it is necessary to monitor 433 foetuses electronically, but this figure may, in truth, be as low as 240 or as high a 2,167.

The study concluded that

> In the light of the evidence now available it is our view that there can be little justification for the use of continuous electronic foetal heart rate monitoring without the facilities to assess foetal acid-base status (foetal blood sampling) when a foetus is thought to be compromised.

There is, therefore, no evidence to support the use of these procedures in normal physiological labours, although there may be a case when the labour shows clear signs of difficulty for either the mother or the baby.

One of the side effects of EFM is the way in which it is deskilling the midwives. At one time all labours were monitored by midwives using a Pinard stethoscope. It looks like a small ear trumpet and by listening with it the midwife is able to detect any impending problems. It is common for women to be asked to have a period of 20 minutes monitoring upon admission to hospital despite the evidence showing that this *increases* mortality. If you are not happy about being immobilised on your bed, with a buckle strapped across your stomach, you can state that you would prefer to be monitored by the midwife with a Pinard.

A problem with electronic foetal monitors is that they sometimes go wrong. If the midwives are not confident in the accuracy of the machine it is better for you to ask for your labour to be monitored by the midwife with a Pinard, or even a Sonicaid (a hand-held electronic monitor). If a machine cannot be trusted it is better off in the cupboard.

In many hospitals EFM also involves fitting a foetal scalp electrode to the baby's head (or bottom if the baby is breech). It means that your waters will have to be broken, if they have not already done so, in order to attach the foetal monitor to the baby's head. This is done with a variety of clips, one of which resembles an S-shaped needle, it is attached to the baby's scalp, just underneath the skin, by a screwing motion. Research has shown that following the attaching of a foetal scalp electrode the baby's heart rate increases to a maximum level for up to ten minutes afterwards. It has been suggested that this response is a sign that the babies are not too happy about this procedure and as they are not able to cry in utero they are displaying their distress by reacting in this manner.

Studies have also shown that using foetal scalp electrodes increases the risk of scalp infections and bruising and is believed to have contributed to the severity of neonatal jaundice. No one seems to be bothered by the possibility of foetal scalp electrodes increasing the risk of the baby contracting HIV or AIDS from an infected mother. In those areas where they believe that a high proportion of the population is HIV+, foetal scalp electrodes should not be used.

Electronic foetal monitoring has been shown not to work and obstetricians are beginning the acknowlege this. They are not, however, abandoning the foetal monitor. As Dr Norman Davies, a research fellow at King's College said,

> In an ideal world the machines would not be necessary. But in this country we are desperately short of trained midwives and a woman in labour will often have several different people looking after her. In these circumstances, it's safer to have a continuous record of what's happening. The big advantage of the electronic monitors is the trace, the hard copy that shows us what's happening.

In other words foetal monitors are better than no midwife at all, and a hard copy is the evidence they want should any mother decide to sue them in the event of a poor outcome. The fact that research has shown that obstetricians are not very good at interpreting foetal monitoring tracings does not seem to abate their enthusiasm.

An American paediatrician, writing in the *Journal of the Royal Society of Medicine*, pointed out that in his hospital in 1986 the Caesarean section rate was 30 per cent, and many of the Caesareans were the direct and exclusive result of monitor tracings. He went on to suggest 'why not turn off *all* the monitors? They do not prevent death or suffering regardless of the level of perinatal risk. They do not reduce workloads or costs in obstetrical units. And they do not prevent litigation.' What he did not mention was that they *do* help to cover up serious midwifery shortages. Heaven forbid that money should be spent employing more midwives, far better to spend it on a nice shiny machine which does not work.

Your rights

You have every right to refuse to be monitored with an electronic foetal monitor, to carry out monitoring against your expressed wishes is an assault.

EPIDURAL ANAESTHESIA

Epidural anaesthesia is the most effective method of pain relief for childbirth and it has been described by some members of the medical profession as the Rolls Royce of anaesthesia. It is given by an injection of a drug epidural bupivicaine into the epidural space in a woman's spine. It is a skilled operation which requires an anaesthetist to carry it out, although midwives are allowed to top up the drug during labour. It has been shown to provide satisfactory anaesthesia in 80 per cent of women, but fails in about 5 per cent; in a further 5 per cent anaesthesia is unilateral (on one side only) or a segment remains unblocked. A few women (1–2 per cent) feel that they have not properly experienced the birth.

One of its great advantages is during a Caesarean section; one can only marvel at the quick recovery of women who have had Caesarean sections with an epidural. It enables the mother to be awake during the birth of her baby, providing her with a memorable and happy experience. In the more progressive hospitals fathers have been admitted to the theatre and been able to share the experience with their partner.

When the epidural works properly you will find that you are completely numb from your waist down. For any woman who has a very painful and exhausting labour an epidural is wonderful, but many women feel that they ought to book an epidural and enjoy their labour by doing *The Times* crossword. A study by Barbara Morgan found that those women who had no drugs for the relief of pain expressed greater satisfaction than those women who had epidurals and 16 per cent of those that had epidurals were less than satisfied with the experience (*British Journal of Obstetrics and Gynaecology*, Vol. 91, 1984).

Little is known about the long-term effects of epidurals but following the public attention given to a mother who was paralysed and in a coma as a result of an epidural, Health Rights received letters from 70 women who described their experiences. One of the major complaints was backache, although the medical profession claims that backache is a common complaint following childbirth and cannot be attributed to epidurals. Many of the women had very serious headaches and for some of them the headaches continued at intervals for years. Some of the women complained about tingling sensations in their limbs or areas of numbness. Had there been adequate research into this technique we would now know whether any of these conditions were a direct result of epidural anaesthesia and how many women it affects each year.

In the short term, it has been shown that there is a systematic tendency for women to be more likely to be delivered with instruments, although it is possible to allow the epidural to wear off towards the end of the labour so that the woman can push the baby out without assistance.

Epidurals also allow doctors to 'drive' the uterus at far higher levels than would be physiologically possible, by winding the oxytocin drip up to high levels. The increased pain this causes is masked by the epidural.

Apart from the medical defence societies no one knows how many epidurals go wrong. In one year the Medical Defence Union settled 285 cases out of court. This has to represent the tip of the iceberg as large numbers of complaints never get as far as legal action, let alone a court. In 1989 a hospital in Cumbria withdrew its booked epidural service because of the numbers of legal cases it had to deal with. Had there been a proper evaluation of this widely used procedure following its introduction we would now be in a better position to judge the risks.

Some women have been told that epidurals are completely safe and do not affect the baby. They do, and what is more they can affect the baby for some considerable time after the birth. Rosenblatt *et al* in their study of the effects of epidurals on the baby have shown that

> Visual skills and alertness decreased significantly with increases in the cord blood concentration of bupivacaine, particularly on the first day of life but also throughout the next six weeks. Adverse effects of bupivacaine levels on the infant's motor organisation, his ability to control his own state of consciousness and his physiological response to stress were also observed. . . . Immediately after delivery, infants with greater exposure to bupivacaine in utero were more likely to be cyanotic (imperfect oxygenation of the blood, the babies have a blue tinge) and unresponsive to their surroundings (*British Journal of Obstetrics and Gynaeology*, Vol. 88, 1981).

One problem women have had with epidurals is that they have booked into a hospital believing that they would have one only to find that the anaesthetist is not available. They have then had to labour without one or have to wait a long time until one was set up.

If you want an epidural for the birth of your baby you will need to find a hospital that does a great many epidurals (the more experience they have the better). Find out how many resident anaesthetists they have and how many women have had epidurals in the last year.

If you book an epidural and then at the last moment you decide you do not want it, you have every right to refuse. Some women who after signing a consent form decided not to have an epidural were told that they could not withdraw their consent. You have the right to withdraw your consent at any time; anyone misleading you in this way and continuing with the treatment runs the risk of being sued for assault.

EPISIOTOMY

It is performed in the interests of mother and child with all the good intentions in the world but with little evidence that in fact it benefits either. However, it has a number of well established undesirable side effects (Michael House, consultant obstetrician, 1981).

The systematic use of episiotomy is not justified (World Health Organisation, 1985).

For the last 35 years or so it has been fashionable to carry out episiotomies. In this procedure the woman's perineum is cut as the baby is about to be delivered. By 1978 55 per cent of women had episiotomies during childbirth and if you were a first-time mother the figure was 70 per cent.

Obstetricians confidently claimed that episiotomy prevented prolapse (without any evidence to support such a claim), prevented tearing, healed better and prevented stress incontinence (e.g. sneeze and you pee involuntarily). Research evidence shows how wrong they were. (A prolapse is a condition in which the uterus (womb) drops as a result of a weakening of the supporting muscles.)

Episiotomy is a procedure which has been vigorously criticised by the majority of the user groups for many years; like so many obstetric interventions it had not been properly evaluated before its widespread introduction. In 1983, however, a midwife, Jenny Sleep, published her findings of a randomised controlled trial of episiotomy (*British Medical Journal*, Vol. 289, 1984).

She compared two groups of women; one group had the standard procedure of liberal use of episiotomy to try and avoid tears and the other group was not given an episiotomy unless it was really necessary. They were clled the 'liberal' group and the 'restricted' group. She found that the liberal group had episiotomy rates of 51 per cent but the restricted group's rates was 10 per cent. 1,000 women participated in the trial.

Overall, she found that the restricted policy resulted in less maternal trauma, more intact perinea and an earlier resumption of their sex lives than the group which had the routine episiotomy. Although the trial found that there were two cases of severe trauma in the women in the restricted group, it was stressed that because of the small numbers this could have occurred by chance; and only a very large trial will reveal whether this is a true risk.

One interesting finding from this trial was that the restricted policy resulted in substantial savings in staff time and suture materials. If the results were to be extrapolated to the whole of England and Wales, the adoption of a restricted policy would save an estimated 10,000 hours of staff time and £65,000 worth of suture materials.

In view of the findings of this trial you should find out what the policies are in the maternity unit of your choice, and ask your midwife what *her* episiotomy rates are. If they are over 10 per cent for the hospital or the midwife, either find another unit or be on your guard.

It is important, however, to realise that there are circumstances when episiotomy is necessary, for example, a forceps delivery. Getting yourself into a squatting position for the birth will help avoid an episiotomy or a tear, and if the midwife is urging you to *push*, rather like a cheer leader at a baseball match, ignore her. It is not necessary to push your baby out with all your might: not only are you likely to over-exert yourself but you are putting additional strain on your perineum at the very time when it needs time to be able to stretch sufficiently to allow your baby to come into the world gently. Push is a word that should rarely be used in a delivery room.

FORCEPS DELIVERY

Forceps were invented during the 16th century by Dr Peter Chamberlen, a surgeon. For the next hundred years his family kept their design secret, thus ensuring a very lucrative income. As Jean Donnison says in her book *Midwives and Medical Men*

It thus gave the doctor or surgeon an addition advantage over the midwife (to whom custom did not allow the use of instruments as an accepted part of her practice) and so further enhanced the position of men.

Thirty years ago an alternative was first used in Britain, Malmstom's obstetric vacuum extractor. This instrument has more or less replaced forceps in most other parts of Europe. It is only in Britain, North America and Australasia that forceps remain as the instrument of first choice in difficult deliveries.

In an article in the *British Journal of Obstetrics and Gynaecology* (May 1989) Drs Chalmers and Chalmers comment

> Outsiders looking in on our speciality must regard it as some-what bizarre that the instrument selected to assist a woman to give birth vaginally apparently depends more on the language spoken by her obstetrician than anything else.

They go on to consider the costs to women of the professions continued use of forceps.

> Assuming that about 50,000 women will require instrumental vaginal delivery every year, the continued use of forceps as the instrument of first choice results, every year, in about 12,000 unnecessary pudendal blocks and other forms of regional anaesthesia for delivery, about 10,000 women unnecessarily experiencing moderate or severe pain during childbirth, 5,000 more women with severe perineal or vaginal trauma than there need be, and 3,500 women suffering unnecessarily from severe pain for several days after delivery.

Forceps are used to assist a woman who has problems delivering her baby, and at that point you are in no position to engage in a protracted argument about using a vacuum extractor instead. But you can take action *before* you go into labour. Find out whether the hospital uses vacuum extractors; if not, you can ask them what steps they are taking to ensure that their doctors are properly trained in their use. If the hospital does not use vacuum extractors you can book into another hospital which does, or book yourself a domino birth, GP unit or home birth. This will reduce the chances of needing assistance with the birth.

INDUCTION AND ACCELERATION

In the early 1970s induction and acceleration became very fashionable so that large numbers of women were admitted to hospital to have their babies delivered on a specific day. Those who came into hospital too early often found that instead of suggesting that they go for a walk, go back home or wait patiently they, too, were induced or had their labours accelerated.

In 1974 the Oxford Consumer Group did a report on women's views of maternity care, this was then taken up later by Oliver and Louise Gillie in *The Times*. In 1976 Jean Robinson, the then Chair of the Patients' Association wrote an article in *The Times* exposing what was happening and questioning the wisdom and validity of induction and acceleration. The Scottish AIMS group had also carried out a survey of women's views which criticised the excessive use of this procedure. Since then the induction and acceleration rates have come down, but not by much.

Obstetricians protest that they do not carry out inductions in order to rush off to their golf course, but they do perform them to fit in with their schedules. Private patients suffer higher rates of inductions because that is one way of guaranteeing that the consultant will deliver the baby. Unlike midwives, many consultants are unwilling to turn out when you go into labour; much better to have you go into labour when it suits them.

A study by Macfarlane showed that the smallest numbers of births occur on Sundays with the maximum on Tuesdays, Wednesdays, Thursdays or Fridays. There are fewer births on Christmas Day and Boxing Day than on any other day of the year. Other public holidays also have low birth rates (*British Medical Journal*, Vol. I, 1979). In other words, women are often induced and accelerated to fit in with the routines and schedules of hospital staff. The best interests of the babies takes second place.

The most common procedure for inducing labour is to break the waters, set up an oxytocin drip and await developments. Many units also use prostaglandin pessaries, which are considered better for women with an unripe cervix. Because oxytocin is a powerful drug the staff will have to watch you carefully. Unfortunately, instead of ensuring that there is a midwife in constant attendance the majority of hospitals attach women to an electronic foetal heart monitor; even though the studies show how inaccurate and unreliable these machines are. It results in women being immoblised on a bed and having little to do or think about except their labour and what is happening. Many women find inductions much more painful than normal labour and the majority of women will request pain relief.

If it is suggested to you that you should have an induction or an acceleration, you should ask the staff why is it indicated in your case and what alternative methods are available. Some women find that the staff have not taken into account the fact that they have a long menstural cycle; they are recommending an induction because the baby is overdue while the woman is arguing that this is not the case. The routine use of ultrasound has reduced the numbers of babies being induced because they are overdue and there is evidence that anyway the interventions made no difference to the outcome. It is reasonable, therefore, for women to have the choice in whether or not they are induced for reasons of post-maturity.

There are many legitimate reasons for induction and acceleration: pre-eclamptic toxaemia (the mother would have protein in the urine), diabetes, high blood pressure, or the distress of the baby.

You should ask the staff to justify their proposals and if you are not satisfied with their reasons you have every right to refuse. You could ask for a second opinion. If they suggest that the baby should be delivered because of some complication affecting it, you could ask for the advice of a paediatrician on whether or not the baby would be better delivered at this time.

Inductions are rarely carried out in home births and used much less frequently in GP unit births.

PETHIDINE

One of the most common methods of dealing with pain in labour in British hospitals is to give the woman an injection of pethidine. Although a powerful narcotic, in a study carried out by the NCT over 70 per cent of women found it an ineffective pain-reliever. It is, however, very effective at keeping women quiet!

Midwifery textbooks suggest that the initial dose should be 150 to 200mg and 100 or 150mg for every repeat dose. In America, however, they are becoming more and more concerned about the long-term effects of drugs in labour on the babies and they have been using 50mg. Doris Haire in her article 'Drugs in labour and birth' describes how a well-controlled investigation by John Morrison, an obstetrician at the University of Mississippi, revealed that one of every four infants of mothers who received only 50mg within one to three hours before delivery required resuscitation at birth. For this reason many American midwives often administer the drug in smaller doses, such as 25mg or 12mg.

If you find that the alternative pain relief methods (below) are not working and you feel you need some drugs, you can ask the staff to give you a much smaller dose.

You have an absolute right to refuse drugs if you do not want them. Anyone who gives you a drug without your consent, or against your expressed wishes, leaves themselves open to a charge of assault.

The alternative methods of pain relief that you could try are:

• walking around or changing position, perhaps getting on to your hands and knees if you are uncomfortable lying on your side (you should not be lying on your back: it can be very bad for you and the baby).

• Having a warm bath or a shower. Michael House, a consultant obstetrician, reported that when he asked women who had had three or more children for their most successful form of pain relief, they said that having a warm bath was far more effective than drugs. He is now trying to instal more baths in the delivery rooms in his hospital.

- Hot compresses on your perineum or a hot water bottle on your back if you have a 'backache labour'
- Massage.

If a midwife tells you that you cannot have any drugs because it is too late, don't despair and think that the midwife is unfeeling and vindictive. What she probably means is 'You can't have any drugs now because the baby is going to arrive within the next twenty minutes or so and the drugs will affect the baby as well as you.' Raise three cheers and try to relax because your baby is about to arrive. The end is in sight!

All the drugs given to you during labour get through to the baby; if you are given drugs late in your labour those drugs will be in the baby's body at birth. A baby's liver is not sufficiently developed to deal with these very powerful drugs and it may be some days before the baby's body clears the drugs from its system. Those women who have droopy, sleepy babies who do not feed very well are often women who have received a large amount of drugs during labour, or within a few hours before the birth.

Recent research indicates that women who receive pethidine are at increased risk of having a baby who will develop cancer by the age of ten. These risks are very small, but avoidable. As pethidine is so ineffective one wonders why its use continues?

PUBIC SHAVING

There is no indication for pubic shaving or pre-delivery enema (World Health Organisation, 1985).

The practice of shaving pubic hair began because some women had lice and shaving was one way of getting rid of them quickly. It was also claimed, without any evidence, that pubic shaving prevented infections. The practice, like most obstetric practices, soon started to be used on everyone; and even when women with lice became rare, pubic shaving still continued, to such an extent that it became one of the rites of admission to hospital.

In 1922 Johnson and Sidall showed that pubic shaving was unjustified because it caused more infections than it prevented (it was the first randomised trial in perinatal medicine). A succession of studies since then were all ignored. In 1980 Mona Romney published research showing that shaving 'increases patient discomfort without reducing infection or improving healing. We believe that perineal shaving is an unjustified assault and should be abandoned'.

Unfortunately, many midwives have taken little notice of the research and now carry out 'partial shaves' – no doubt in the fond hope that they will only cause a 'partial infection'. In 1984 a survey of 208 maternity units was undertaken, it found that in 49 per cent of units hardly anyone was shaved, in 24 per cent of units almost everyone was shaved and in 25 per cent of units the practice was somewhere in between.

Your rights

You have an absolute right to refuse to have pubic shaving. To carry it out without your consent or against your expressed wishes is an assault.

SYNTOMETRINE

This form of management was developed as part of the response of the profession to the problems of postpartum haemorrhage. As happens so often with developments in obstetrics, all mothers came to be treated in the same manner, irrespective of the degree of risk. Those who have a normal first and second stage could be allowed to complete the process normally. With a physiological third stage (i.e. without syntometrine) there is time for the mothers to explore her baby and possibly put it to the breast while the attendants wait quietly for the signs of separation of the placenta (Chard and Richards. *Benefits and Hazards of the New Obstetrics*, p 120).

Syntometrine is a drug which is commonly used in the active management of the third stage of labour – that is, the stage between the complete birth of the baby and the delivery of the placenta and membranes. It consists of 5 units of syntocinon (a synthetic form of oxytocin) and 0.5 mgm of ergometrine. The syntocinon causes the womb to contract within two or three minutes of the injection and the ergometrine causes a further and sustained contraction some seven minutes after the injection. It is usually given with the birth of the baby's shoulders. The midwife or doctor wants to deliver the placenta before the action of the *ergometrine* which could trap it. The cord is clamped immediately to stop the baby receiving a dose of syntometrine and the placenta is delivered by controlled cord traction as soon as the first contraction caused by the *syntocinon* is felt.

The drug was developed to help prevent postpartum

haemmorhage, the risk of which increases with the numbers of deliveries. Before the 1950s when the majority of women had their babies at home, women expecting their seventh, eighth or more babies were at increased risk of haemmorhage and there was little the midwives could do about it. Having found a drug that helped, the well-developed principle, 'if it's good for a few then it must be even better for everyone', was employed. Without any proper evaluation, the use of syntometrine became a routine in British hospitals. Many women are often unaware that it has been done as they are concentrating on delivering their new baby.

A recent randomised controlled trial to evaluate the risks and benefits of active management of the third stage of labour reported that postpartum haemorrhage was 5.9 per cent in the group allocated to active management and 17.9 per cent in the physiological group. A great deal of debate has followed. Unfortunately, the physiological group included women who had previous third-stage problems, oxytocics to induce or augment labour, large doses of narcotics, epidurals or forceps deliveries. The study was also being conducted by midwives who were not accustomed to practising physiological management, although the researchers have acknowledged that subsequent changes in the protocol of physiological management, and the increased confidence of the midwives, may have contributed to some real improvements in outcome; but there was still a need to conduct a randomised controlled trial of active versus physiological management of the third stage in setting in which physiological management is the norm.

If you have had a normal physiological labour and delivery without the use of drugs you may wish to ask the midwife not to use syntometrine unless you start bleeding. If, however, you have had an induction or accelerated labour, as well as other drugs in labour, the midwife will want to use syntometrine as the drugs have already perverted normality. Having had oxytocin (the drug used to induce and accelerate labour) you are already running almost double the risk of having a postpartum haemorrhage.

If you do decide not to have syntometrine it is most important to ensure that no one pulls on the cord. There have been cases of women refusing syntometrine and the doctors hauling on the cord. This action has caused some women to have acute inversion of the uterus, a very dangerous condition.

12

POSTNATAL CARE

DISCHARGE FROM HOSPITAL

A mother may discharge herself and her baby from hospital at any time. A early discharge is sometimes looked upon with disfavour by the hospital staff who may require the mother to sign a form stating that she has discharged herself against medical advice.

One Health Authority, however, took this one step further and required mothers to sign the following:

> I understand and acknowledge that as my discharge from hospital was not foreseen by them (sic) I do not hold the Community Midwifery Service of Croydon Area Health Authority responsible for providing their usual maternity follow-up facilities for me.

A health authority has a statutory obligation to provide the services of a midwife for up to at least ten days after the birth. Croydon AHA's action above was illegal – they subsequently withdrew this form after pressure from AIMS.

A mother is under no obligation to sign a discharge form should she not wish to do so. If she does decide to sign it she should be aware that officialdom often views an early discharge against medical advice as irresponsible. If you subsequently become involved in a complaint or litigation you may find your early discharge being interpreted in that way. You will not be able to challenge this unless you have signed the discharge form and also *added your reasons* for taking that decision.

When you are discharged from hospital the staff should tell the local midwives so that they can visit you up to ten days, but longer if you or your baby are not well. If a midwife does not arrive on your doorstep the day after you arrive home from hospital, then the following day you should telephone the Supervisor of Midwives at the hospital, tell her that a midwife has not yet arrived and ask if the community midwives have been informed.

At one time women were required to stay in hospital for at least ten days after the birth of their baby, but over the years that time has been severely reduced. With the present staff and bed shortages hospitals are encouraging women to go home as soon as possible. If, however, you do not feel well enough to return home, or feel that the circumstances are not right you can insist on remaining in hospital for a further period.

HOME HELPS

A newly delivered mother has the right to expect a home help for up to ten days post-natally. The Social Services Department has a legal obligation to provide one (maternity cases take priority – NHS Act 1977, Schedule 8, para 3(i). Some Local Authorities means-test applications, but the charge varies from area to area, and some Local Authorities make no charge at all for this service (NHS Act 1977, Schedule 8, para 1(2), 3(2). Applications should be made to your local Social Services Department. Your local Health Visitor or GP will be able to give you the address.

Some mothers are told that they have to have special circum-stances which justify the provisions of a home help – otherwise they will not be eligible. This is false. A request for a home help from a newly delivered mother *must* be treated as a priority. If you have twins, or more, have had a Caesarean section and have little or no support at home you should be using this service. Women are being denied this service because they do not know it is available, and those who do make a request are told that all the home helps are busy with geriatric care and there is no one to spare. Contact AIMS if you fail to get a home help allocated.

INFANT FEEDING

The decision whether to bottlefeed or breastfeed your baby is yours. When bottlefeeding was the norm a breastfeeding woman was looked upon as something of a peculiarity, and many were required to draw the curtains around their beds to shield the rest of the mothers from this strange woman. Since then breastfeeding has been recognised as far better for the baby, and bottlefeeding mothers may find people questioning their decision not to breast-feed. There are many reasons why women choose not to breastfeed.

- They have no confidence in their ability to breastfeed.
- They have had problems breastfeeding and decide to give up and give the baby formula food.
- They (or their neighbours, friends or family) have had previous bad experiences with breastfeeding and they want to avoid these this time.
- They will be returning to work very soon and want the baby established on the bottle before they do so.
- They find breastfeeding distasteful.

Respecting and supporting the rights of individuals to come to a decision about their care appears to be a concept which has yet to be grasped by many members of the midwifery and medical professions. It is also apparent that it is not enough for health professionals to exhort women to breastfeed: they must in addition provide the good quality care to help women to do so without major difficulties. Women who wish to breastfeed often have problems which result from being given wrong information or from not having access to skilled help.

Women who wish to breastfeed need to have the right to do that successfully, without sore nipples, severe engorgement, an inconsolable baby, or any of the other problems which result from a lack of good support.

Having argued in the 1970s and 1980s for women to be able to breastfeed if they wanted, AIMS is now concerned about the rights of women who wish to bottlefeed. It is not in the interests of either the mother or the baby to coerce her into a method she does not want. Even though her baby is receiving formula food the mother will still be giving her baby vital contact, cuddles and love. Women who choose to bottlefeed need access to information, too, about the correct use of formula; they need access to clean, safe, water and facilities for sterilisation, and they may need financial help to buy the supplies and equipment required.

Although 65 per cent of women begin to breastfeed only 40 per cent are still doing so at six weeks. It is striking that women from poorer backgrounds choose to breastfeed less often and, when they do, they stop sooner than more affluent women. So the health-giving and cost-saving benefits of breastfeeding are lost to those who may need them most. There are a multitude of reasons given for why women stop breastfeeding sooner than they would like. One common problem is the huge variety of advice given by midwives and doctors in the early postnatal period. Breastfeeding has to be learned and it can easily be disrupted. Another is women's loss of confidence in their own bodies, and the resulting anxiety that they are not able to produce enough milk.

In many units babies were commonly given 'top-ups' either of water soon after birth, or milk supplements in the belief that the mother's milk was inadequate. This activity disrupted the establishment of breastfeeding and many mothers gave up. It is still not uncommon for hospitals to recognise that breastfeeding mothers need to feed on demand, yet insist that the 'demand' feeding is done at specific times.

If you are breastfeeding your baby it is important that your baby remains with you. You can then ensure that your baby is not given additional bottles of water or formula feed. You have the right to insist that your baby remains at your side. Some babies are taken into Special Care for 'observation', and in some hospitals 'rooming-in' is not available. There is no evidence supporting the separation of healthy mothers and babies, and there is research evidence which shows that separating mothers from their babies led to an increase in the subsequent risk of child abuse and neglect among socially deprived, first-time mothers.

Thanks to the activities of Baby Milk Action, and Edwina Currie MP, the majority of British hospitals no longer give women free samples of formula feeds to take home with them. It was shown that this activity resulted in many women being tempted to give their baby a bottle; having done that they were at risk of disrupting breastfeeding, and subsequently give up because of the problems. Following this ban the formula feed companies looked for other markets. In some areas they now give the health visitors packets of infant food for 'weaning' (which is quite unnecessary: babies can be weaned on to normal food which has been mashed up for them). The baby milk companies are now vigorously promoting their formula feeds in the Third World; as a consequence babies in Africa, Asia and the Far East are being bottlefed and are suffering and dying as a result.

The largest offender in this new sales drive is Nestlé, as a result of their aggressive marketing methods in the Third World, Baby Milk Action launched a renewed boycott of their products in 1989, in an attempt to draw public attention to the ethically questionable activities of this particular multinational.

In 1988 a Joint National Breastfeeding Initiative was launched to promote and encourage breastfeeding in Britain. It is a joint effort between three UK breastfeeding support organisations in co-operation with health workers and their professional organisations. Further information can be obtained from the Joint Breastfeeding Initiative, Alexandra House, Oldham Terrace, Acton, London W3 6NH. Tel: 081-992-8637 or 081-690-0506.

If you are having problems breastfeeding and want to continue you can ask your midwife or health visitor for advice. You can also contact a number of organisations specifically concerned with breastfeeding: the National Childbirth Trust, which has breastfeeding counsellors in most areas, the Association of Breastfeeding Mothers or the La Lèche League. You could also find out whether there are any breastfeeding mothers in your own neighbourhood and discuss your problems with them. If you are in hospital and having problems many hospitals have a lactation sister who specifically concerns herself with helping women breastfeed. You could also find out whether there are any experienced breastfeeding women on your or nearby wards, have a word with them. There is nothing like personal experience. Very few women are incapable of breastfeeding, many give up because of conflicting advice, lack of support or loss of confidence. It is a question of accurately identifying the problem and then taking what is the best action for you.

When breastfeeding is fully established it is very easy indeed, you don't have to carry around armfuls of equipment; you don't have to heat the milk to the appropriate temperature, and you don't have to spend any time at all sterilising the equipment. When baby needs a feed, you put him/her on the breast. The British, however, are rather ambivalent in their attitudes to women breastfeeding in public places. A survey by the Joint Breastfeeding Initiative of 1020 restaurant managers revealed that 17 per cent had a mother-and-baby room, 11 per cent had another room available and 72 per cent expected the women to breastfeed in the toilet. I don't eat in a toilet and I would consider anyone who did to have a rather disgusting habit. It is, therefore, even more disgusting to expect a small baby to have his/her meal there. If you are having a meal in a restaurant and the baby needs feeding then s/he should be fed too. It is not necessary to expose vast areas of breast, it is perfectly possible to breastfeed discreetly and the more women do it the more acceptable it will become. You have every right to feed your baby wherever you choose and, apart from expressing disapproval, there is little anyone can do about it. It is not you who has the problem but those who disapprove, they need to examine why they feel the way they do.

The campaign by the Joint Breastfeeding Initiative to ensure adequate facilities for mothers with small babies is most welcome, but I do have some reservations about breastfeeding being hidden away. It is a perfectly natural human activity and it is time that our culture moved away from the attitude that breasts have only one function best illustrated on page three of the gutter press.

POSTNATAL DEPRESSION

Postnatal depression is a common complication following childbirth. It affects 10 to 15 per cent of all postnatal women and up to

8 per 1,000 will experience a severe psychotic form. It is now so common in British hospitals it has almost achieved the status of a pandemic and there appears to be a general acceptance that one will get it. Interestingly, the rates are very much lower in women who have home births.

Theories about the causes range from an hormonal imbalance to psychoanalitical interpretations. Whilst it is possible that the three-day 'baby blues', where women suddenly burst into tears and have a good cry for no apparent reason, can reasonably be considered to be caused by an hormonal imbalance it is difficult to reconcile that with the woman who at two or three months becomes depressed. The psychoanalitical viewpoint focuses on women who have had painful periods in adolescence, didn't get on with their mothers, dislike housework, suffered a recent bereavement, etc, etc.

Ann Oakley has pointed out that many women with postnatal depression have had high-technology births and were socially vulnerable. Significant factors were housing problems, not being employed, having a 'segregated' marital role-relationship and not knowing much about babies before becoming a mother.

In our 'work' orientated society women's work in the home it does not carry a very high status. Many have the shock of being totally responsible for a small vulnerable being and finding them-selves alone and confined to the house, probably in an area where they know very few people. The public image of a young mother is one of a well-dressed capable person in an immaculate house with an immaculately turned-out child. The reality is very different and it is time that we stopped playing this charade and acknowledged that bringing up small children is often hard grinding work, with little mental stimulation and often an isolating experience. Very few of us have our parents and families nearby and so often we know very few people in our own neighbourhood. The positive side of having children is that it can offer an opportunity to mature and grow, they are often wonderful to be with and give us a great deal of love and fun.

A significant proportion of those who have had a high technology birth are probably trying to think positively about it. What is remarkable is not why do women get postnatal depression, but why do some women *not* get postnatal depression.

For some women postnatal depression creeps up on them and it may be some time before they recognise what they are suffering. Feelings of lethargy and tiredness, unable to cope with the house-hold chores, unwillingness to go out, feelings, of sadness, sudden panic attacks and difficulty with sleeping; many may find them-selves in tears for part of the day. The sheer hard work of looking after a small baby twenty-four hours a day is enough to induce that in the fittest of people, so it is sometimes difficult to recognise that one may be suffering from postnatal depression.

So, what can one do about it? Many women who feel unhappy about the birth can be helped to talk about their feelings and discuss the causes. In those who feel strongly it can be very therapeutic for them to write a letter of complaint and address these issues. I believe that a great deal of postnatal depression is connected with suppressed anger. As women we are conditioned not to get angry and to hide our real emotions. For many, the experience of a technological birth can be traumatic. Many women feel that they are taken over, it is not unusual for women who have had very traumatic births to complain that they felt they were subjected to medicalised rape. Taking action and doing something about the experience can help recovery considerably.

Health visitors will visit from ten days after the birth to offer their services, which you may find extremely helpful. If you find them less than helpful you can decline to see them, or if one specific individual is unhelpful you can ask for another health visitor to attend. If some time has elapsed since the birth, and you feel in need of some support and advice, you could give the health visitor a call and discuss your feelings with her. Your GP can be helpful too. In some circumstances GPs will prescribe anti-depressants, and these may be helpful in some cases. Check with your pharmacist that the prescribed drugs are not addictive, many of them are and in the 1970s and 1980s huge numbers of women become addicted to Valium as a result of enthusiastic over-prescribing by GPs.

If you are not certain that the advice you are being given is right for you then seek other advice, the ways of dealing with postnatal depression are not written in stone and there are many alternatives. It is a question of accurately identifying what is wrong and taking appropriate action. Once in a while a woman will approach a GP who does not believe that postnatal depression even exists, so she will have to deal with that problem either by finding another GP or by seeking support and help elsewhere.

Katerina Dalton believes that postnatal depression is caused by hormonal imbalances and has developed a treatment. Whilst it has clearly helped many women there are those who are very critical of it and feel that the issue is not quite that simple. Research by William Hague, a research fellow at the Middlesex Hospital, has revealed that 6 to 9 per cent of mothers have postpartum disturbances due to low thyroid hormone levels. In mild cases there is no treatment and the condition rectifies itself. In some severe cases treatment would be indicated. Many women have low blood pressure or anaemia postnatally and it is worth having this checked too. At least if you know what is causing the problem you will be half way there in dealing with it.

Helpful organisations

Meet-a-Mum Association. 58 Malden Avenue, S. Norwood, London SE25 4HS

National Childbirth Trust. Alexandra House, Oldham Terrace, London W3 6NH

Association for Post-natal Illness. 25 Jerdan Place, Fulham, London SW6 IBE

POSTNATAL EXAMINATION

Six weeks after giving birth you should have a postnatal examination. This is usually done by your GP, although research shows that not everyone has this check. It also shows that 45 per cent of women would have preferred having a female carry out the examination. If you feel this way there is no reason why you cannot approach your community midwife and ask her to do it.

The purpose of the six-week examination is to check that your uterus has returned to normal, and that you and your baby are fit and healthy. If you have any worries, either about your own health or that of your baby, this is a good time to discuss it. The question of future contraception will also be raised, but many women prefer to make their contraceptive arrangements with their local well-women clinic or family planning clinic.

The internal examination will check the size of the uterus, which by now should have shrunk back to somewhere near its pre-pregnancy size. The traditional vaginal examination by a doctor to establish complete involution is viewed by some to be unwarranted. It is considered unlikely to yield any useful information and is often carried out at the expense of more useful items, such as discussing contraception and breastfeeding, how the woman feels, and how the baby is settling into the family.

If you have any vaginal soreness or still having problems with an episiotomy, you can discuss what to do about it with the midwife or GP. Research shows that a proportion of women have problems with their episiotomy for some time postnatally. One should not 'grin and bear it', if you still have problems by the six-week check up this is the time to make a fuss about it and find out what action can be taken to rectify it.

Some women will be suffering from stress incontinence. Suffered

by around 8½ per cent of women between the ages of fifteen and
sixty-four years. They accidently leak urine when they cough,
sneeze, jump or laugh. It is often accepted as a consequence of
having a baby and believed to be caused by weakened pelvic floor
muscles or the results of high forceps delivery, Caesarean section,
epidural anaesthesia, or from having an indwelling catheter for
more than twenty-four hours. The condition often responds very
well to exercise but you can discuss this with your midwife/GP or
health visitor. A referral to an obstetric physiotherapist is often very
helpful.

The quality of postnatal checks varies considerably around the
country. Your GP will be paid £11.25 for this check whether he
spends a couple of minutes asking you how you are or half an hour
giving you a complete check and the opportunity for a full
discussion.

SPECIAL AND INTENSIVE CARE BABY UNITS

Occasionally babies are unwell following the birth and they are
taken to the special or intensive care baby unit for treatment. While
the staff in the majority of these units try very hard indeed to
involve parents in their baby's care there are times when some
parents very intimidated by these units and feel that control is
taken from them.

One cannot give consent for treatment for another person, but as
the parents of the child you can give assent, which allows the staff
to treat your baby. In theory you should be told what treatment is
necessary and what is being given, in reality parents are often
unaware of much of what happens in special care and intensive
care units.

You have the right when your baby is admitted to be informed of
precisely why s/he is being admitted, and what treatments they
propose to carry out. Those parents who are concerned about the
misuse of ultrasound are often unaware that a baby in an intensive
care unit may be subjected to an ultrasound scan every day. If the
baby has had a traumatic delivery the use of scans may be appropriate, you should establish why they are carrying out these
examinations and decide whether or not you wish them to continue.
Many special care and intensive care units carry out research, so
you can ask what research is being done and decide whether or not
you want your baby involved in such a programme.

A recurring problem for mothers who have babies in special care
is the issue of breastfeeding. Many women want to breastfeed their
babies and often find that the unit is some distance from where
they are. This can be a major obstacle when the mother has had a

difficult confinement and is herself recovering, perhaps from a Caesarean section. If the arrangements for breastfeeding are not working, you can ask to see the senior nurse or midwife in the unit and discuss the problem with her. If she is not helpful then you can ask the see the Director of Midwifery Services.

Parents sometimes find that their baby has been taken to a unit in another hospital so that they have additional problems of access. If this has happened see if arrangements can be made for you to transfer too. If you are having to travel to a unit you may be able to claim the costs of travelling (see page 11), and if you have other children at home you can ask Social Services to provide a home help to give you additional support and assistance (see page 121).

THE LOSS OF A BABY

A miscarriage is the spontaneous loss of a baby before the twenty-eighth week of pregnancy. This is often referred to in medical terms as a spontaneous abortion, and women often get very upset when they have lost a wanted baby within this period and the doctor refers to it as an abortion. Abortions, in the mind of the public, are associated with the deliberate termination of a pregnancy.

A stillbirth is the birth of a baby after the twenty-eight week of pregnancy which neither breathes, nor shows any other sign of life following complete expulsion from the mother. A neonatal death refers to a baby which, having been born alive, dies within the first month after birth, and a perinatal death refers to a death which occurred just prior to, during and up to twenty-eight days after the birth.

Miscarriage

Miscarriage in early pregnancy is not uncommon and is known to occur in around 15 per cent of all pregnancies. A small proportion of women will repeatedly miscarry and very little is known about the reasons for this. If, however, you are a woman who has suffered repeated miscarriage, and have had more than three, you can ask for additional tests to be done to determine the reasons, but very often this will reveal nothing. This is often the most difficult thing for the parents and the professional attendants to accept, and the enthusiasm for doing these tests varies from obstetrician to obstetrician.

In Britain, when a baby dies before twenty-eight weeks there is no legal obligation to issue a death certificate, and there are no statutory obligations about what happens to the baby's body. Many parents find this attitude deeply upsetting, but have been helped by supportive clergymen who have conducted a special memorial service for them. In practice most babies will be cremated by the hospital and some hospitals will make special arrangements. A few hospitals hold a service before cremating the remains. If you are not happy with the hospital arrangements you can take the baby with you and make your own; although some hospitals are not particularly happy about parents doing this. If you arrange for the baby to be cremeated you will need a statement from the hospital saying that the baby was less than 28 weeks and showed no signs of life. You should also understand that because the foetus is so small there will probably not be any ashes for you to scatter. If you decide to bury your baby in the garden do remember that you may well move house.

It is not routine for health visitors to visit parents who have suffered a miscarriage, but if you feel you need someone to talk to and need some support and advice you can contact your local health visitor and ask for a visit. Unfortunately, women who miscarry are often left to get over it on their own and are often unsupported.

There are many women who are recommended to remain in bed following a threatened miscarriage after bleeding has occurred in early pregnancy. While one may wish to stay in bed for a period and should be free to do what one feels inclined to do, there is no scientific evidence to show that this makes any difference at all to the chances of maintaining the pregnancy.

Stillbirth and neonatal death

In recent years the needs of the parents following a stillbirth have been recognised and many hospitals have made special arrangements. A photograph of the baby is usually taken and kept in the case notes. If, sometime in the future, you feel you would like to have it you will be able to do so. Not every woman wants to hold her baby after the birth, some women take a few days to come to terms with what has happened and then ask to see the baby. This is often particularly important for women who have given birth to babies who were born with some abnormality. Sensitive midwives will wrap and dress the baby and will stay with the mother and explain the nature of the abnormality and the possible reasons for it. Women who have seen their babies in these circumstances have said that their images of what the condition was like were far worse than the reality, and they were helped considerably by being able to see their baby.

At one time the death certificate, for babies over twenty-eight weeks, was called a *Certificate for Disposal*, and Hugh Jolly, a paediatrician, waged a lengthy campaign (joined in the latter stages by AIMS) to have it changed to a *Death Certificate.*

Parents are often too shocked after the death of their baby to make decisions, and they are sometimes asked to agree to the burial of the body before they are ready. If the baby is more than twenty-eight weeks old the hospital can arrange the burial, if the parents wish. It is usually buried in a communal grave. Unfortunately some parents who enquired where their baby had been buried discovered that the cemetery staff could only point to a general area of the cemetery, and were unable to pinpoint the exact spot. You do not have to agree to the burial or cremation of your baby immediately. You can, if you wish, take your baby's body with you and make your own arrangements for a funeral.

Some hospitals provide a small chapel where the baby is taken and the parents will have the opportunity of spending some time with their baby grieving and saying goodbye.

In some circumstances the hospital may wish to carry out an autopsy (also called a post-mortem) you do not have to agree immediately, you can take a little time to think about whether you want it done. It does have the advantage of possibly identifying the reasons why your baby died. Although there are occasions when babies die for no identifiable reason. You are not entitled to see the autopsy report, although your GP will get a letter from the hospital describing the results, you can either discuss this with the GP or arrange an appointment with the consultant to talk about it with him/her. If you particularly wish to see the autopsy report you could give your consent to the autopsy on condition that you receive a copy of the full report.

If you are concerned about the reasons for your baby's death you could visit the local coroner and ask him to conduct an enquiry. He has the right to conduct an enquiry into any death which occurs in his area.

Sometimes when parents have lost a baby they believe that they had poor medical or midwifery care and blame their attendants. This belief may or may not be justified but it is often not helped by the response of the attendants to the tragedy. It may be that the staff are as upset as the parents but they may not be able to convey their feelings and present an image of not caring or they may seek to avoid contact.

It is not always possible for care to be perfect all of the time, staff shortages, errors of judgement and lack of resources sometimes play a part in a tragedy. For the parents it can be very therapeutic to make an effective complaint and receive full and honest answers to their questions. In some circumstances, particularly when it becomes clear that the authorities are being less than honest, the parents feel that the only course left open to them is legal action.

Legal action serves two purposes, obtaining the case notes and obtaining monetary recompense. The majority of parents are horrified by the idea of financial payment for the loss of their baby, but many are, by this stage, so incensed by the behaviour of those who should be helping them that they take this course of action. If health authorities were honest about the train of events and gave immediate access to the case notes the vast majority of these cases would go no further. As it is, the anguish of parents is prolonged by a lengthy complaints system sometimes followed by even lengthier legal action. Such events often prevent parents grieving properly and continuing with their lives.

Helpful organisations

Stillbirth and Neonatal Death Society (SANDS). 28 Portland Place London W1N 4DE 071-436-5881

Miscarriage Association. PO Box 24 Ossett West Yorkshire WF5 9XG, 0924-264579 (weekday mornings)

13

BIRTH IS NOT AN ILLNESS!

In April 1985 I was invited to attend a World Health Organisation conference in Fortaleza, Brazil. The conference followed a similar one held in Washington USA in November 1984 which I co-chaired with Professor Roberto Caldeyro-Barcia, the past President of the International Federation of Obstetricians and Gynaecologists.

The Brazilian conference had been organised because people all over the world were becoming increasingly anxious about the over-medicalisation of childbirth. The purpose of the conference was to discuss the issues, consider the best way of confronting the problems caused by the proliferation of obstetric technology, and make recommendations for good practice.

There were sixty-two conference delegates from Europe, Canada, the USA and Central and South America. They included obstetricians, paediatricians, midwives, statisticians, epidemologists and three lay representatives of whom I was one.

Over a period of five days the delegates met and considered 'appropriate technology for birth'. Although at times, there were wide-ranging views about appropriate technology, there was also a surprising amount of agreement.

On the final day the delegates itemised the recommendations on which the conference agreed and twenty-six of them were summarised and published by the WHO in June 1985.

In March 1987 I, together with Christine Rodgers (the Hon Vice Chair of AIMS), were invited to a conference in Italy and discovered that Piera Maghella Alvarez, the founder of MINA, an Italian childbirth group, had taken the WHO recommendations and published a list of the fifteen most appropriate for her country.

The idea was so exciting that we brought the Italian version back to Britain and promptly published a Britain version which is published here under the title *Birth is Not an Illness*! The leaflet is printed on yellow paper (a symbol in Italy for women) and is available in A2, A3 and A4 sizes from AIMS. Their objective is to have these leaflets and posters put up in every antenatal clinic, GP surgery and Community Health Council offices in Britain.

The idea has been taken up in seven other countries, France, Brazil, Ireland, Finland and Sweden. In the USA the magazine *Childbirth Alternatives Quarterly* has published a version. In this way it is hoped that the WHO recommendations will receive international attention and the professionals will begin to focus on the validity of what they are doing.

BIRTH IS NOT AN ILLNESS!

15 recommendations of the World Health Organisation

The following are some of the recommendations of a joint Inter-regional Conference for Birth, held in 1985 and arranged by the Regional Officers for Europe and the Americas of the World Health Organization.

The recommendations are based on the principle that each woman has a fundamental right to receive proper prenatal care; that the woman has a central role in all aspects of this care, including participation in the planning, carrying out and evaluation of the care; and that social, emotional and psychological factors are decisive in the understanding and implementation of proper prenatal care.

- The whole community should be informed about the various procedures in birth care, to enable each woman to choose the type of birth care she prefers.
- Information about birth practices in hospitals (rates of Caesarean section, etc.) should be given to the public served by the hospitals.
- There is no indication for pubic shaving or a predelivery enema.
- Birth should not be induced for convenience. No geographic region should have rates of induced labour over 10 per cent.
- Artificial early rupture of the membranes, as a routine process, is not scientifically justified.
- There is no evidence that routine intrapartum electronic foetal monitoring has a positive effect on the outcome of pregnancy. Electronic foetal monitoring should be carried out only in carefully selected medical cases (related to high perinatal mortality rates) and in induced labour. Countries should carry out investigations to select specific groups of pregnant women who might

benefit from electronic foetal monitoring. Until such time as results are known, national health care services should abstain from purchasing new monitoring equipment.

- Pregnant women should not be put in a lithotomy position during labour or delivery. They should be encouraged to walk about during labour and each woman must freely decide which position to adopt during delivery.
- During delivery, the routine administration of analgesic or anaesthetic drugs, that are not specifically required to correct or prevent a complication in delivery, should be avoided.
- The systematic use of episiotomy is not justified.
- There is no justification in any specific geographic region to have more than 10 to 15 per cent Caesarean section births.
- There is no evidence that a Caesarean section is required after a previous transverse low segment Caesarean section birth. Vaginal deliveries after a Caesarean should normally be encouraged wherever emergency surgical capacity is available.
- The immediate beginning of breastfeeding should be promoted, even before the mother leaves the delivery room.
- The healthy newborn must remain with the mother, whenever both their conditions permit it. No process of observation of the healthy newborn justifies a separation from the mother.
- Governments should consider developing regulations to permit the use of new birth technology only after adequate evaluation.
- Technology assessment should be multidisciplinary and involve all types of providers who use the technology. The women, on whom the technology is used, should be involved in planning the assessment as well as evaluating and disseminating the results. The results of the assessment should be fed back to all those involved in the research as well as to the communities where the research was conducted.

The full set of recommendations is published by the Regional Office for Europe of the WHO, and is available from AIMS.

14

COMPLAINTS PROCEDURES

There are endless reports which recognise the dissatisfaction that exists with maternity care. Perhaps we have the care we deserve; until we start speaking out about matters in need of improvement, we will continue to have it.

Some 650,000 babies are born in Britain each year. This means that around half a million parents will use the maternity services offered by their local health authority. Some of those parents will not be satisfied with the care they have received and some of them will wish to complain about it. Many, however, will not complain. A common response is often along the lines of: 'Well this is going to be my last baby, so I won't need to go back there again,' or 'Well, I don't want to get anyone into trouble,' or 'If I complain then they will take it out on me the next time.'

The latter anxiety is a very real one, parents often find that details of their complaint have been written on their files and some of the staff act accordingly the next time. Unfortunately, the woman's response to this is to try her hardest to be nice to the staff concerned, a response which often reinforces their behaviour. If, however, the mother makes it clear she is not going to tolerate any nonsense this time, the staff often behave themselves and act in a more professional manner.

It is my view that not only should people with justifiable complaints go ahead and complain, but they should consider it a duty to other mothers. If you have something serious to complain about you should do so; otherwise your silence will ensure that the next mother who sees that particular, doctor, midwife, health visitor or other staff member is almost guaranteed to suffer the same kind of treatment. Unless it is made clear to the staff that certain behaviour and attitudes are unacceptable they will continue to behave or practise badly, for there will be nothing to curb them or make them think again.

The therapeutic effect of making a formal complaint should not be overlooked. Many parents find it very helpful to sit down and write about their experiences from the beginning. It often produces many tears, but it is very common for the parents to comment that even though they cried a great deal they felt very much better afterwards.

The complaints procedures are very complicated. The following information is general and will, one hopes, give you an idea of the rules and conditions that apply, and broadly what you steps you can take.

MAKING A COMPLAINT

If you feel that your complaint is fairly minor, you should find the senior person on duty and tell them about it as soon after the incident as possible. If, however, you feel that the complaint is of a more serious nature, (or that your verbal complaint was not taken seriously), then it is essential that you put your complaint in writing. *Always* keep a copy. Occasionally, complaints 'get lost' and if that should happen to you you have no evidence that you actually made a complaint, or to whom it was sent if you have not made a copy.

TO WHOM SHOULD THE COMPLAINT BE SENT?

Complaints about GP care

These should be sent to the Family Health Services Authority. You will find the address in the telephone directory under Family. In Scotland write to the Primary Care Division of the Health Board; in Northern Ireland, Central Services Agency.

The FHSA must receive the complaint within *thirteen weeks* of the incident. In Scotland the time limit is still *six* weeks but there are proposals in hand to increase the time limit. (Note: If you are complaining to the FHSA you will have to allege a breach of the regulations, otherwise the FHSA will not investigate your complaint.) You should, therefore, write your letter of complaint and make the following statement in the final paragraph:

> I would appreciate it if you would investigate these complaints about Dr . . . who was, I believe, in breach of his/her terms of service.

If you are too ill to face writing your complaint to the FHSA within the deadline, send the FHSA a letter stating that you intend complaining once you have recovered and will write a full complaint in the near future. This will ensure that your complaint is registered and you will not be disqualified because of failing to meet the time restrictions.

There is an appeals system. Both you and the GP have a right of appeal and you do so by writing to the Secretary of State of Health as soon as possible after the hearing.

If you have a complaint about the *administrative action* taken in your complaint, or if you are dissatisfied with the way the FHSA handled an informal complaint, you have grounds for asking for an Ombudsaman investigation.

If your complaint to the FHSA was upheld and the doctor was found guilty, the FPC is required to inform the DH who will report him to the General Medical Council (GMC). In which case you are no longer considered by the GMC to be the 'primary complainant' and, therefore, you will not be allowed copies of any transcript, nor will you be allowed to listen to all the evidence. There have been occasions when the complainant was not aware that their case had been forwarded to the GMC. It is necessary, therefore, for you to report the doctor to the GMC yourself and inform them that you are to be considered the 'primary complainant'.

Complaints about hospital care

Write to the District General Manager (Scotland: Unit General Manager). You can obtain his address from the hospital in which you had your baby or from the Community Health Council (Scotland: Local Health Council, Northern Ireland: District Committee).

The complaint should be received within one *year* of the incident. Outside that time limit you can still put in a complaint, and it will be investigated, but the official complaints procedure need not be followed.

Complaints about junior medical staff (doctors) should be sent to the District General Manager with a copy to the consultant obstetrician, the Chairs of the Regional Health Authority and the District Health Authority. In Scotland write to the Unit General Manager with a copy to the Health Board.

Complaints about consultant obstetricians should be sent to the District General Manager with a copy to the Chairs of the Regional Health Authority and District Health Authority. In Scotland write the Unit General Manager with a copy to the Health Authority.

Complaints about midwives should be sent to the District General

Manager with a copy to the Supervisor of Midwives (Scotland: Unit General Manager)

Complaints about health visitors and nurses should be sent to the District General Manager with a copy to the Director of Nursing Services.

PROFESSIONAL MISCONDUCT

If, having complained to the appropriate authorities locally and your complaint also involves professional misconduct, you can either make a complaint to the professional bodies following the local investigation, or you can make a direct complaint to the professional bodies in the first place. If your complaint involves circumstances in which more than one individual is involved, you should consider whether you have a complaint against the other staff too.

For midwives, nurses and health visitors you can write to the English National Board (Scotland: Scottish National Board, N. Ireland: N. Ireland National Board) sending a copy of your complaint for information to the United Kingdom Central Council for Nurses, Midwives and Health Visitors.

Each country has its own National Board which investigates complaints. If they find there is a case to answer they will then refer it to the UKCC's Professional Conduct Committee. It is this committee which will hear the charge and if they consider it sufficiently serious can strike the nurse, midwife or health visitor off the list or take various disciplinary actions. The UKCC is a body which takes its role of maintaining standards very seriously indeed, unlike the General Medical Council which appears to spend its time avoiding taking action against doctors.

Complaints about all medical staff (junior hospital doctors, GPs and hospital consultants) which involve professional misconduct should be sent to the General Medical Council.

If you are making a complaint to the General Medical Council you should send copies of your complaint to the doctor about whom you are complaining (because if your complaint is rejected by the Preliminary Screener the doctor (or anyone else) is not informed that there has been a complaint made against him/her).

Copies of the complaint should also be sent to the Chair of the Regional Health Authority (Scotland: Health Board, Northern Ireland; Health and Social Services Board) and District Health Authority (Scotland: Health District, Northern Ireland: Health and Social Services District). See page 141 for further information about the General Medical Council.

With any complaint that you are making you should always let others know what is happening, otherwise you may find that the complaint is dealt with quietly and no one else is aware of what has been going on. Therefore, with all complaints send copies to:

- Chair, Regional Health Authority (Scotland: Health Board, Northern Ireland: Health and Social Services Board)
- Chair, District Health Authority (Scotland: Health District; Northern Ireland: Health and Social Services District)
- Chair, Community Health Council (Scotland: Local Health Council; Northern Ireland; District Committee)
- Chair, Association for Improvements in the Maternity Services.

If the complaint is a serious one you should also send a copy of it to your local MP, so that he is aware that all is not well in his area.

The professional bodies concerned are as follows:

- General Medical Council, 44 Hallam Street, London W1N 5LH
- United Kingdom Central Council, 25 Portland Place, London W1M 3AF
- National Board for Nursing, Midwifery and Health Visiting for Scotland, 22 Queen Street, Edinburgh EH2 1JX
- Welsh National Board for Nursing, Midwifery and Health Visiting, 13th Floor, Pearl Assurance House, Greyfriars Road, Cardiff CF1 3AG
- National Board for Nursing, Midwifery and Health Visiting for Northern Ireland, RAC House, 79 Chichester Street, Belfast BT1 4JE

If you still feel dissatisfied with the response you have had to your complaint you can take your complaint further. There are a number of stages involved within the Health Authority (depending on the nature of your complaint) so you should make it clear (in writing) that you are dissatisfied with the findings and enquire to whom you should direct your appeal, and ask for details of the options open to you. Copies of this letter should also be sent to the same people to whom you sent copies of your complaint.

If you are dissatisfied with the findings of the General Medical Council, the UKCC or the various National Boards you can ask for a judicial review. You must ask for a judicial review within three months of the final decision and you can apply for legal aid for this.

GOLDEN RULES

- Decide what are the most important items you wish to complain about and stick to them; do not wander off the point.
- Write your letter of complaint clearly and number each complaint

you wish to have investigated. Having numbered each item separately it is then much easier to write back thanking them for their reply and pointing out that you have not had a reply to item number x.

- Do *not* write pages of detail, carefully discussing each minute incident. Not only will the reader be bored stiff by the end, they are unlikely to read more than the first few pages properly. Fifteen pages of closely written text is daunting even for those who are sympathetic to your case. So try your best to restrict the length of your letter of complaint (aim at maximum of four pages of A4).
- Be sure to mention the good care you received and any kind and considerate people who dealt with you (otherwise you run the risk that they will dismiss you as a 'complainer').
- Do be clear. You may know what you are writing about but it is sometimes not at all clear to the reader. If you are quoting previous correspondence enclose a copy of the relevant letter (preferably use a highlighter to identify the particular passage you are writing about).
- If you are invited to a meeting to discuss your complaint, under no circumstances go alone. Take someone with you who has experience of dealing with bureaucracies (some CHCs provide assistance; check that they have some good calibre people, some CHCs can be very unhelpful). If you cannot find anyone from a supporting organisation then at least take your partner or a family friend.

GENERAL MEDICAL COUNCIL

Serious complaints about doctors (GPs, hospital doctors) are referred to the General Medical Council. This body was set up to 'protect' the public from incompetent doctors, but in reality its major role appears to be limiting the numbers of complaints against doctors. Around 1,000 complaints a year are sent to the GMC and up to three-quarters are rejected before any kind of hearing.

Any complaint to the GMC is first considered by the 'Preliminary Screener'. His role is to consider the complaint; if it is serious enough it is referred to the Preliminary Proceedings Committee.

The Preliminary Screener decides which cases go forward. He is appointed by the President and the past President, Sir John Walton, appointed himself to this role. The current President, Sir Robert Kilpatrick, has continued this practice. This means that if he rejects a case there is no higher authority to appeal to. Sir Robert Kilpatrick as President of the GMC is hardly going to uphold an appeal against a decision made by Sir Robert Kilpatrick the Preliminary Screener! In order to deflect some of the criticism of this practice the President has chosen a lay screener to look at those cases which he has rejected. It will be interesting to see how effective the lay screener will be at critically examining these rejected complaints. The GMC still gives no information about rejected complaints, where they come from and what they are about. It is, therefore, impossible to compare the rejected cases with those which have gone forward.

The procedures at the GMC compare very unfavourably with those of the UKCC which has a committee which considers whether or not complaints should be referred to their Professional Conduct Committee.

Jean Robinson, one of the lay members of the GMC (nominated by the Association of Community Health Councils in England and Wales and appointed by the Privy Council) has described the GMC's activities as 'a farce, albeit a smooth running and gentlemanly farce'. She was so concerned about the GMC's activities she wrote a book, *A Patient Voice at the GMC.* Anyone making a complaint to the GMC should read this superb exposé first.

Comparatively few complaints from the public get to the Preliminary Proceedings Committee; the bulk of cases come from the police (drunken driving, shoplifting) and from the FPCs (the DH can refer cases where the GP has been found guilty following an FHSA hearing). This means that the majority of clinical cases heard involved GPs. There is no obligation upon Health Authorities to refer hospital doctors to the GMC following a serious complaint; hospital doctors are almost untouchable.

Those cases which allege serious professional misconduct are heard in public and the burden of proof required is equivalent to that required in a court of law.

The GMC does not usually carry out primary investigation of the cases itself; unlike the United Kingdom Central Council for Nurses, Midwives and Health Visitors (the equivalent body to the GMC) which has to investigate every complaint and is very open about its activities.

The GMC is amazingly secretive about its hearings. At a hearing in 1986 where a GP involved with an anaesthetic death the GMC would not allow any details of the charges to be given until the doctor stepped into the room to answer them. The Press were informed that there was a case against Dr. . . . which involved anaesthesia. What they were not told was that the doctor was being charged with serious professional misconduct that resulted in 'a woman dying because he had left her alone and unconscious following an operation'.

It is not even possible to obtain transcripts of a public hearing held by the Professional Conduct Committee. The GMC only releases transcripts to those who have been involved in the case provided they pay a hefty fee (around £400 per day's hearing) for the privilege.

This attitude compares very unfavourably with the UKCC, which not only allows access to the transcripts of the hearing for researchers, but also sends copies to the relevant health authority, to help ensure that they are aware of the problem and can take steps to prevent it happening again. The UKCC has also contacted user groups and informed them of a hearing which will be of interest to them.

If you are dissatisfied with the findings of the General Medical Council you can ask for a judicial review. This must be done within three months of the final decision and you can apply for legal aid for this.

THE OMBUDSMAN

If, having exhausted the local complaints procedures you still feel dissatisfied you can take your complaint to the Ombudsman (the Health Service Commissioner). There are, however, limitations on the kind of things he can investigate. He cannot investigate matters involving medical treatment (clinical judgement), nor the activities of the Family Practitioner Committee, unless the FPC dealt with the case informally or that they failed in some administrative way, e.g. failing to tell you what the complaints procedure is or failing to tell you the outcome of their deliberations.

A condition of the Ombudsman's investigations will be an agreement that you do not plan to take legal action.

There is a time limit for complaints to the Ombudsman. The complaint should reach him within a year of the incident, so do not allow the health authority to delay in replying to your complaints. Even though you may be outside the time limit, it is still worth putting in the complaint. In serious cases, the Ombudsman has discretion about whether or not to investigate a late complaint.

Although the Ombudsman was set up in order to have an independent examination of parents' complaints the procedures used to evaluate the complaint are weighed against the complainant.

After the Ombudsman receives your letter of complaint, he shows it to the staff at the hospital who comment on it. You are not allowed to see the comments the staff have made, and there have been instances where the staff make up incidents to support their colleagues and diminish your case. If they can show you to be an unreasonable, awkward, person that will reduce the strength of

your complaint. Staff who were not even present at the incident
will be brought in to substantiate what has been said.

The Ombudsman then considers the case and makes his decision.
He neither allows you to see what the staff have said about you nor
gives you the opportunity to comment. It is a very unsastisfactory
system: because you do not find out what has been said until you
have received his judgement, you are in no position to refute it
until it is too late.

Recently, however, there have been some interesting developments. In February 1987 Mrs A attended Rutherglen Maternity Unit,
Glasgow, for her first antenatal appointment (the Ombudsman's
report does not identify individuals). She was seen by a consultant
obstetrician who was accompanied by students. The experience led
her to complain to the Ombudsman that the consultant did not
obtain her prior agreement to the presence of students; that he did
not introduce himself, or speak to her directly, but merely pushed
her into position for the examination and made a series of sarcastic
remarks, that the Health Board's initial response to her letter of
complaint was unsatisfactory, and their replies were unnecessarily
delayed.

Mrs A was already apprehensive when she attended for her first
examination, because she had been warned that the internal examination would not be very pleasant. At the clinic she was attended
by two 'nurses' (even the Ombudsman has not learnt the difference
between nurses and midwives), one of whom was a student and
they were both very nice. A doctor came and took blood and then
the consultant arrived with two medical students, who stood and
watched while she was being examined.

Mrs A was not asked for her permission for the students to be
present even though she thought she ought to have been. She was
already being examined when the consultant and the students
arrived, and she did not want to cause a scene.

The consultant obstetrician's response to this complaint was that
as this was a teaching hospital it was 'self-evident' that medical
students would be present and he did not normally ask a patient if
she objected to students being present, but assumed that she
would know that they would be there, and assumed that she had no
objections. He also acknowledged that he has not changed his
practice since she made her complaint.

The Ombudsman found that 'the consultant made too sweeping
assumptions claiming that it was self-evidence that students would
be present as this was a teaching hospital'. He saw no reason why
ordinary patients should know that, and expected the consultant to
be sensitive to a patient's apprehension about an internal examination; and criticised the Health Board for failing to inform women,

and seek their permission, about the presence of medical students. Apparently the Board is now reviewing the wording on their appointment cards.

Mrs A also complained that the consultant failed to introduce himself, failed to address her directly and made sarcastic remarks about her to the students. She said she had her legs bent up and parted for the examination but the consultant kept roughly pushing her legs further and further apart, even while speaking to the students. Needless to say she felt very embarrassed. She accused the consultant of 'showing off to the students, at my expense' and that she 'might as well have been a piece of furniture'. One of his remarks was 'look at this, what a disaster', apparently referring to the fact that her womb was tilted. He also made a series of comments to the effect that 'women are all like that, they are all just a disaster, they have always got something wrong'. She could not believe what she was hearing and as the examination progressed she grew redder with embarrassment and anger. She said there had been other remarks too, which she could no longer recall, but she remembers being struck by their personal and sexist nature.

The consultant said that he did not recall the appointment with Mrs A, but admitted that he did not routinely introduce himself. He felt that he would explain what he was going to do, and denied emphatically that he would have pushed her legs apart. He said he would merely have asked her to lift up her knees. In order to put patients at their ease it was necessary to approach them with confidence and as she had an acutely retroverted uterus the outcome could have been 'disasterous' had he not corrected it. He could not recall remarking that her womb was a 'disaster' and that 'all women were disasters', and being sarcastic would be a waste of time as one of his medical students did not have a perfect grasp of English. He felt that if Mrs A felt aggrieved she should have raised the matter with him at the time.

One of the medical students, who could not remember the incident, felt the consultant would usually chat with his patients and could not recall any of the remarks, but she did think that 'the consultant was of the old school; very good but extremely strict and not as careful of women's feelings as the newer generation of doctors'. The other medical student thought the consultant was friendly, quite extroverted and enthusiastic about his work. He had never known the consultant make sarcastic remarks about patients.

The senior nurse generally supported the consultant but did comment that one group of student midwives had told her inform- ally that they did not like the consultant's manner. To which she replied that 'he was of a different era and that bedside manner and language used could differ greatly from doctor to doctor, and had emphasised the consultant's clinical excellence. She said the consultant was a big man, and she wondered if some women found that a little frightening. She suggested that perhaps the consultant's bigness and loudness worked against him.

The midwifery sister was similarly ambiguous and described the consultant as one of the older style doctors, with a somewhat brusque manner. She herself had told him she would send him to charm school for a week.

The staff midwives also sought to justify the consultant's behaviour but acknowledged that the students had accused him of being intimidating and rude to patients, but one staff midwife pointed out that they had been unused to working with consultants. (A hint perhaps that dealing with rude, arrogant, consultants was par for the job.)

Two of the three student midwives who had been present did not recall the incident but they all felt it likely that the complaint was justified. One student described the consultant as very abrupt with patients and never appeared particularly interested in them. It was a case, she said of 'get them in, on the couch and out again'. She described him as 'very brash, very rude'. One of the students in describing a similar incident to this commented 'I don't think people should be put through that.' They explained that overall the consultant did not usually introduce himself, he spoke very little to his patients and would not always explain what he was going to do. The third student midwife said that she would never forget the incident and was completely 'floored' by it.

A student nurse in the clinic who was present at the examination said she vaguely recalled the consultant making a joking remark to the medical students about women's anatomy always having problems and not being built to the same standard as men's.

The Ombudsman found that:

> The consultant's manner may well be perfectly acceptable to many patients. But I believe that he should be sensitive to the possibility that towards others, and particularly towards patients in their first pregnancy there may be a need to modify and soften his approach and manner. I believe he failed to take sufficient account of that need in the complainer's case, with the result that she was embarrassed and offended. To that extent I am critical of him, and uphold this complaint.

Mrs A also complained about the unsatisfactory and delayed response from the Board, the reply took seven weeks, she felt that she expected an apology and instead got the distinct impression that she was being told off, for example:

It is normal practice to ensure adequate training that students be present at examinations. If, however, a patient does not wish students to be present and this is indicted at the time then her request will be complied with. You will appreciate however that if all patients adopted this attitude then students would not be able to get training essential to them. Fortunately the great majority of patients accept this situation and raise no objections.

The administrator concluded the letter with 'May I suggest that any future attendances at clinics where students are present and you still have objections you should indicate so at the outset.'

The delay in replying had been caused mainly by the consultant giving the administrator 'absolutely no information' and no specific comments had been made about the incident, because the consultant did not remember it. The consultant had said that it was not his 'normal practice' to behave in the way alleged and the administrator had to accept this. (One of the problems complainants have with the complaints system is the failure of administrators to deal properly with consultants who behave in this manner.)

The administrator felt that Mrs A was looking for a straightforward apology but he could not do that without the consultant's agreement and clearly that was not going to be forthcoming. The delay was caused because he was trying to extract an apology from the consultant, when he proposed offering the woman an apology the consultant refused to be associated with it so the apology could only come from the Board. In which case he should have approached the Board.

Mrs A's response to the administrator's letter was to write stating that 'You yourself have a bad attitude and you are just as pigheaded as the doctor in question.'

The Ombudsman upheld her complaint about the delay and agreed that the letter had a chiding tone, but he found that 'I consider the personal remarks she made about the administrator were uncalled for and inappropriate.'

He concluded:

While I am sure that the consultant would not intentionally upset a patient. I hope that my report will give him cause to consider how his manner may appear to others.

The Health Board asked the Ombudsman to extend to Mrs A their apologies for the shortcomings he identified and that they would be writing to her directly with an apology. The Scottish Home and Health Department plans to issue a circular which would provide guidance to health boards on the need to ensure that patients are willing to co-operate in medical education.

The Ombudsman, in this case, accepted what the woman said about the consultant's attitude, although he clearly felt that his behaviour was not meant unkindly. What would have been the response if Mrs A had not had a group of student midwives who were prepared to stand up and acknowledge that this particular obstetrician is a bad-mannered, sexist, bore?

It was clear from the Ombudsman's gently chiding criticisms that the consultant was unmoved by this complaint.

In December 1989 the Select Committee called three representatives of the Health Board to answer questions at the House of Commons. During the course of a long interview with the administrators the Chair of the Select Committee expressed the view that 'It does display a monstrous attitude to a patient' and when the administrators tried to play down the incident,

> I think it was said somewhere in the papers that this was possibly his method of relaxing the patient, obviously it had the very opposite effect. The Chairman intervened 'A disaster area!'. . . . It is a pity he is not here and we could see if we could make him feel reassured in a similar manner.

At this hearing the administrators assured the Select Committee that Rutherglen Maternity Unit, Glasgow, has now given more information to women about their rights when medical students are present.

The length of time from initiating a complaint to an investigation by the Select Committee is very long, but it does at least provide a means of calling a health authority to account for the behaviour of its medical staff. If more women made formal complaints about rude obstetricians significant changes would soon be achieved.

TAKING LEGAL ACTION

Legal action is not a course to be undertaken lightly and few parents are willing to take a legal route to resolve their complaints. It is the experience of AIMS that the vast majority of complainants want no more than to find out the truth of what has happened to them and want to be assured that their experience will not be repeated and, where justified, receive an apology.

The medical profession, on the other hand, seems to hold the view that every complainant is a potential litigant and takes every means possible to dissuade them from continuing with their complaint. Such action frequently forces the parents into taking the very action the profession is seeking to avoid.

From the 1st November 1991 patients will have a right to apply to see their case notes, but this right does not apply to notes made before that date. Access to those notes will still require the patient to take legal action. When legal action has been taken many Health Authorities will only agree to release the case notes to a solicitor, or a doctor nominated by your solicitor, with the proviso that you do *not* have access to them. You should not agree to this; it may be very important indeed that you see the case notes. One mother, however, made a postnatal appointment at the hospital and when her case notes appeared in the pile she walked off and photocopied them. (It is not illegal to take your own case notes and photocopy them.)

If you decide to take legal action, the first thing you should do is find a good lawyer. Do not make the mistake of engaging the nice man who was so efficient at conveyancing when you bought your house, or the young woman who dealt with a case of harassment from your neighbour. What you need to find is a *good medical lawyer* that is a lawyer who is experienced at medical litigation. It is also wise to engage a lawyer who does not live in your area. Very often the lawyers know the obstetrician involved, belong to the same clubs and live in the same neighbourhood. You need someone who does not have the problems of knowing the defendents.

Finding good lawyers is a very real and difficult problem. In his book, *Lawyers can damage your Health*, Michael Joseph detailed the disasters and tragedies that can occur when you engage a lawyer who doesn't know much what he is doing. Quite apart from the idle and negligent ones!

It is also very difficult indeed to change lawyers mid-stream, not only are you faced with trying to identify a good lawyer who would be willing to take on a legal mess, you also have the problem of costs.

The Association for Victims of Medical Accidents is a superb organisation which helps patients who want to take legal action. A voluntary organisation, it will give you advice on sympathetic solicitors in your area.

You should consider applying for legal aid. Though many people fall outside the legal aid provisions, you may be surprised to find you are eligible.

Although legal aid will support some litigants through their legal action, it is entitled to recover the amount granted should you receive an award from the court. You should, therefore, consider what it is you want to achieve, and whether the lengthy proceedings and the constant strain are worth it.

It is worth remembering that the success rates of people who take legal action over medical negligence is very low and inversely proportional to those who take civil action. In other words, in civil actions (for example, suing the local builder) over 70 per cent of litigants win their cases, in medical negligence cases over 70 per cent of defendants (the medical profession) win the cases.

It is clear that judges have considerable problems in objectively assessing cases of medical negligence and are very reluctant to find against the doctors. This means that you must have a very strong case to succeed. Where there is a dispute over clinical judgement, the judge is likely to be very hard to convince. Unfortunately, litigation has little to do with justice and a great deal to do with playing games in court.

It is not only the patients who suffer from this problem. When Wendy Savage, the consultant obstetrician who was accused of negligence by her colleagues, asked the High Court to intervene in her case, the judge (Mr Justice Walton) decided not to do so with the comment that 'as obstetrics was difficult to understand and would involve hours of instruction from the medical profession it would be better if Ms Savage's case was judged by her own profession'. An interesting argument because learned judges do not appear to demonstrate any reluctance or express any difficulty in judging architects, builders or people accused of extremely complex fraud and embezzlement cases. Yet obstetrics, it appears, is too difficult to understand. It has been suggested that as most judges are geriatrics they have an overwhelming personal need to believe in the efficacy of the medical profession and cannot bring themselves to believe that there could be anything seriously wrong with the medical profession.

Having found your lawyer, his/her first action should be to obtain your case notes and any other relevant records (depending upon what your case is about) like X-rays, co-operation cards, nursing notes, etc. Unfortunately, many inexperienced lawyers proceed to obtain medical and legal opinions on your case without first having obtained the case notes.

It is vitally important that your lawyer obtains the case notes at an early stage because they sometimes reveal other instances of negligence or poor care that should also be pursued.

You should also ensure that the qualifications of those who attended you are checked. You may discover that the young doctor who carried out an unsupervised forceps delivery was not qualified to do so without supervision.

You should also consider the non-legal aspects of your case which could properly be investigated by the Health Authority. Often a Health Authority says that as you are taking legal action they will not investigate your complaint. That is not good enough: there is no reason why they should not investigate those aspects which are not subject to litigation and their failure to do so are grounds for a complaint to the Ombudsman.

The role of the midwives is also important. You may have separate actions to take against them, and in the case of midwives you have a controlling body (the United Kingdom Central Council for Nursing, Midwifery and Health Visiting) which takes very seriously any complaint brought to their attention. Unfortunately, the parallel body, the General Medical Council, which is concerned with doctors, is not very interested in user complaints and very few complaints indeed result in the disciplining of the doctor.

CONCLUSION

Though this book is written in the hope that it will arm you to deal with some of the problems that may present themselves, you should not approach the staff assuming that problems will occur. Many midwives and doctors have been very upset when confronted with a hostile woman who, before the poor staff have even said a word, has presumed they are the enemy. If you assume that everyone is lovely you may well find that they are; if you come across the one who is not, that is the time to deal with them.

If you find yourself in conflict with the staff ask yourself one question: what do I really want? Do I want a good birth, or do I want to be nice to the staff? Far too many women give in if there is a difference of opinion because they 'do not want to upset the midwife or doctor'. If there is a choice to be made between upsetting them, and getting the kind of birth you will remember with a warm glow, you will need to decide which has the greater priority for you.

15
STATUTORY AND VOLUNTARY ORGANISATIONS

SUPPORTIVE ORGANISATIONS

Any mother who finds herself meeting opposition to her requests should not, under *any circumstances*, battle on alone. It is important that she seeks help from lay groups who are sufficiently informed to advise her. The following groups are recommended:

Association for Improvements in the Maternity Services
Health Rights (for people in London)
Society to Support Home Confinement

There are innumerable organisations involved with maternity care. The following is a list of those that have been mentioned in this booklet together with some of the other organisations:

Action for Victims of Medical Accidents
Bank Chambers
1 London Road
Forest Hill
London SE23 3TP
081-291-2793
Gives help and advice to those wanting to take legal action.

Active Birth Centre
55 Dartmouth Park Road
London NW5 ISL
071-267-3006
Fax 071-267-5368

Association of Breastfeeding Mothers
131 Mayow Road
London SE26 4HZ
081-778-4769

Association for Improvements in the Maternity Services
Goose Green Barn
Much Hoole
Preston
Lancs PR4 4TD
071-278-5628

Association for Post-natal Illness
25 Jerdan Place
London SW6 IBE
071-386-0868

Association of Radical Midwives
62 Greetby Hill
Ormskirk
Lancs
L39 2DT
0695-572776

Caesarean Support Network
2 Hurst Park Drive
Huyton
Liverpool L36 1TF
051-480-1184

CERES (Consumers for Ethics in Research)
PO Box 1365
London N16 OBW

Community Health Councils
(Usually listed in the local telephone directory under Community)

Health Rights
Unit 110
BonMarché Building
444 Brixton Road
London SW9 8EJ
071-274-4000 x 442/377
Fax 071-737-5521

Independent Midwives Association
65 Mount Nod Road
London SW8 2LP
081-677-9746

Joint Breastfeeding Initiative
Alexandra House
Oldham Terrace
London W3 6NH
081-992-8637 or 081-690-0506

Maternity Alliance
15 Britannia Street
London WC1X 9JP
071-837-1265
Gives help and advice about maternity benefits.

Maternity Defence Fund
33 Castle Street
Henley-in-Arden
West Midlands

Meet-a-Mum Association
c/o 58 Malden Avenue
London SE25 4HS
081-656-7318

National Childbirth Trust
Alexandra House
Oldham Terrace
London W3 6NH
081-992-8637
Fax 081-992-5929

Society to Support Home Confinements
Lydgate
Lydgate Lane
Wolsingham
Bishop Auckland
Co Durham DL13 3HA
0388-528044

Stillbirth and Neonatal Death Society (SANDS)
28 Portland Place
London W1N 3DE
071-436-5881

Special Delivery
34 Elm Quay Court
Nine Elms Lane
London SW8 5DE
071-498-2322

VBAC Information
8 Wren Way
Farnborough
Hants
0252-543250

Wide Awake Club
22 Kings Lea
Heath Charnock
Adlington
Lancs, PR7 4EH

PROFESSIONAL BODIES CONCERNED WITH CHILDBIRTH

Association for General Practice Maternity Care
c/o The Surgery
Temple Sowerby
Penrith
Cumbria CA10 1RZ

Department of Health
Alexander Fleming House
London SE1 6BY
071-407-5522

General Medical Council
44 Hallam Street
London W1N 6AE
071-580-7642
Fax 071-436-1384

Health Service Commissioner for England (The Ombudsman)
Church House
Great Smith Street
London SW1P 3BW
071-212-7676

Royal College of General Practitioners
14 Princes Gate
London SW7 1PU
071-581-6523

Royal College of Midwives
15 Mansfield Street
London W1M OBE
071-580-6523
Fax 071-436-3951

Royal College of Obstetricians and Gynaecologists
27 Sussex Place
London NW1 4RG
071-262-5425

National Perinatal Epidemiology Unit
Radcliffe Infirmary
Oxford OX2 6HE

United Kingdom Central Council
23 Portland Place
London W1M 3AF
071-637-7181
(This replaces the Central Midwives Board)

Each country has its own national board. They are:

English National Board for Nursing, Midwifery and Health Visiting
Victory House
170 Tottenham Court Road
London W1P OHA
071–388–3131

National Board for Nursing, Midwifery and Health Visiting for Scotland
22 Queen Street
Edinburgh EH2 1JX
031–226–7371

Welsh National Board for Nursing, Midwifery and Health Visiting
Thirteenth Floor
Pearl Assurance House
Greyfriars Road
Cardiff CF1 3AG
0222–395535

National Board for Nursing, Midwifery and Health Visiting for Northern Ireland
RAC House
79 Chichester Street
Belfast BT1 4JE
0232–238152

A *MIDIRS Directory of Statutory and Voluntary Organisations relating to Midwifery and Maternity Care in the United Kingdom* can be obtained from the Midwives Information and Resource Service, Institute of Child Health, St Michael's Hill, Bristol BS2 8DJ.

HEALTH RIGHTS

Health Rights is a London-based voluntary organisation working on a broad range of public health and NHS issues. It carries out research; publishes reports and booklets; organises conferences and campaigns; works with a wide range of organisations and agencies.

Health Rights provides advice and information to individuals, voluntary and community groups, health professionals, statutory bodies, and the media. It receives core funding form the London Boroughs Grants Scheme.

Aims and objectives

Health Rights believes that everyone, irrespective of sex, race, class, sexual orientation, age, physical and mental ability, has the right to the health care and treatment they need and the right to health. Health Rights' aim is to promote these basic 'health rights'. It believes they can only be achieved through substantial improvements in the nature, quality and organisation of health services; and through more comprehensive and effective pubiic health measures.

To achieve these aims Health Rights works on a number of key NHS issues to secure specific improvements in health services, and more generally, promotes the need for greater commitment to preventive and public health measures. Further information is available from: Health Rights Ltd, Unit 110, BonMarché Building, 444 Brixton Road, London SW9 8EJ.

ASSOCIATION FOR IMPROVEMENTS IN THE MATERNITY SERVICES (AIMS)

The Association for Improvements in the Maternity Services was established in 1960 after the founder and President, Sally Willington, wrote to a national newspaper about her bad experiences of antenatal care. A deluge of complaints from other women arrived, and AIMS was born.

AIMS' members (parents, midwives, doctors and health professionals) are drawn from all over Britain and Ireland, as well as abroad. There are AIMS contacts throughout the country, which campaign on local issues.

AIMS publishes a quarterly journal which has information concerning campaigns, maternity news, obstetric practices, scientific papers, book and film reviews, readers' letters, members' accounts of their experiences of the maternity services, and current research and developments. The journal spearheads discussion about change and development in the maternity services. It is highly regarded, both by parents – who find it an excellent source of information and support – and by midwives and doctors – who frequently write to AIMS to say that the journal is the best source of information of its kind.

As a campaigning pressure group AIMS has been in the forefront of the childbirth movement in Britain and has provided much of the dynamism for change in childbirth.

In addition to its public campaigning work, AIMS also receives many letters from individual women and couples requesting information and advice, and responds to requests for help as fully as possible.

AIMS has consistently supported the midwife in her role as a practitioner in her own right, who, in normal circumstances, undertakes the care of the mother and baby throughout pregnancy, birth and the period afterwards.

AIMS has campaigned in the past for:

- fathers to be admitted to the labour wards
- a reduction in the routine use of technological interventions such as induction and electronic foetal monitoring
- a severe reduction in the use of routine episiotomy
- a stop to the routine procedures of shaves and enemas

- a randomised controlled trial of chorionic villus sampling

  Some of the current campaigns are for:

- the recognition of childbirth as a normal physiological process
- Health Authorities to make safe and adequate provision for home birth
- a stop to routine ultrasound examination as its safety and efficacy have never been properly evaluated
- a stop to the routine use of syntometrine in labour
- an Office of Technology Assessment so that new technologies in maternity care can be evaluated *before* their widespread introduction.
- a halt to the soaring Caesarean section rates
- that the parents' right to make decisions concerning their own and their baby's care be respected
- the right of mothers to choose to be mobile during labour and to choose the position in which to give birth
- right of access to maternity unit statistical data
- right of access to medical records
- support for a new Midwives Act

Many improvements in maternity care have not come about as a result of professional activity but by the constant pressure and campaigning of user groups.

AIMS believes that parents must have a place to turn for support and encouragement. They need a group whose aims are to campaign to improve all aspects of maternity care, publish and collect information, and further the cause of the parents' right to make informed decisions about their care and birth of their children. Further information from: AIMS, Goose Green Barn, Much Hoole, Preston, Lancs, PR4 4TD, 071-278-5628.

BOOK LIST

AIMS, *Denial of Parents' Rights in Childbirth*, 1983.

Balaskas, J. and Gordon, Y. *Waterbirth: The Concise Guide to Using Water During Pregnancy, Birth and Infancy*, Unwin Paperbacks, 1990.

Balaskas, J. and Gordon, Y. *The Encyclopaedia of Pregnancy and Birth*, Macdonald Orbis, 1988.

Balaskas, J. *New Active Birth: A Concise Guide to Natural Childbirth*, Unwin Hyman, 1989 (revised edn).

Beech, B. *et al. A Commentary on the Report of the Royal College of Obstetricians and Gynaecologists Working Party on Routine Ultrasound Examination in Pregnancy*, AIMS, 1988.

Birth Special Supplement, 'Royal Society of Medicine Forum on Maternity in the Newborn, ultrasonography in obstetrics', Blackwell, 1986.

Borg, S. and Lasker, J. *When Pregnancy Fails* – Coping with Miscarriage, Stillbirth and Neonatal Death, RKP, 1982.

British Medical Association and Royal Society of Medicine, *You and Your Baby*, 1987.

Campbell R. and Macfarlane A. *Where to be Born? The Debate and the Evidence*, National Perinatal Epidemiology Unit, Oxford.

Chamberlain, M. *Old Wives' Tales: Their history, remedies and spells*, Virago, 1982.

Cohen, N. W. and Estner, J. *Silent Knife: Caesarean prevention and vaginal birth after Caesarean*, Bergin and Garvey, 1983.

Comport, M. *Surviving Motherhood*, Ashgrove Press, 1989.

Cronk, M and Flint, C. *Community Midwifery* – A Practice Guide, Heinemann Medical Books, 1989.

Dalton, K. *Depression after Childbirth. How to recgonize and treat postnatal illness*, OUP, 1989.

Donnison, J. *Midwives and Medical Men*, Heinemann, 1988 (revised edn).

Ehrenreich, B. *For Her Own Good: One hundred and fifty years of the experts' advice to women*. Pluto Press. 1979.

Enkin, M. and Chalmers, I. (eds). *Effectiveness and Satisfaction in Antenatal Care*, Heinemann, 1982.

Enkin, M., Keirse, M. and Chalmers, I. (eds). *A Guide to Effective Care in Pregnancy and Childbirth*, OUP, 1989.

Flint, C. *Sensitive Midwifery*, Heinemann, 1986.

Haddad, F. *Journal of the Royal Society of Medicine*, February 1985.

Hall, M. *et al. Antenatal Care Assessed: A Case Study of an Innovation in Aberdeen*, Aberdeen University Press, 1987.

Horwood, J. *Comfort for Depression*, Sheldon Press, 1988.

Inch, S. *Birthrights – A Parents' Guide to Modern Childbirth*, Green Print Merlin Press, 1989 (2nd edn).

Inch, S. *Approaching Birth Meeting the Challenge of Labour*, Green Print, 1989.

Kitzinger, S. *Breastfeeding Your Baby*, Dorling Kindersley, 1989.

La Leche League International, *The Art of Breastfeeding*, Angus and Robertson, 1988 (3rd edn).

Lorenz R.P. *et al.* 'Randomised prospective trial comparing ultrasound and pelvic examination for preterm labour surveillance' *American Journal of Obstetrics and Gynaecology*, 162, 1603–10, 1990.

Macdonald, D. *et al.* 'The Dublin Randomised Controlled Trial of Intrapartum Electronic Foetal Heart Rate Monitoring', 1983.

Medical Defence Union, *Consent and Treatment*, 1974.

Melville, A. and Johnson, C. *Cured to Death: The Effects of Prescription Drugs*, Stein and Davy, 1983.

Maternity Alliance, *Working Parents' Rights*, Maternity Alliance.

Monaco, M. and Junor, V. *The Home Birth Handbook*, Souvenir Press, 1984 (2nd edn).

Moulder, C. *Miscarriage: Women's Experiences and Needs*, Pandora.

Munro, Dame A. *Maternity Care in Action Part 1* – Antenatal Care, HMSO, 1982.

Price, A. and Bamford, N. *Bestfeeding Guide for the Working Woman*, Century, 1984.

Richards, M. 'Perinatal morbidity and mortality in private obstetrics patients', *Journal of Maternal and Child Health*, September 1979.

Renfrew, M., Fisher, C. and Arms S. *Breastfeeding: Getting Breastfeeding Right for You*, Celestial Arts, California.

Richards, L. *Vaginal Birth After Cesarean Experience*, Bergin and Garvey, 1987.

Romney, M. *et al.* 'Pre-delivery shaving: an unjustified assault?', *Journal of Obstetric and Gynaecology*, 1, pp. 33–35, 1980.

Romney, M. *et al.* 'Is your enema really necessary?', *British Medical Journal*, vol 282, p. 126.

Sosa, R. *et al.* 'The effect of a supportive companion on perinatal problems, length of labour and mother and infant interaction', *New England Journal of Medicine*, vol. 303, no. 11, 1980.

Stark, *et al.* 'Short- and long-term risks after exposure to diagnostic ultrasound in utero', *Obstetrics and Gynaecology*, 3, pp. 194–200, 1984.

Tew, M. *Safer Childbirth? A critical history of maternity care*, Chapman and Hall.

Tew, M. 'Is home a safer place?', *Health and Social Science Journal* September 1980.

Wesson, N. *Home Birth – A Practical Guide*, Optima.

Welburn, V. *Postnatal Depression*, Fontana, 1986 (updated).

'Maternity Care in Action', 2nd Report of the Maternity Services Advisory Committee for the Secretaries of State for Social Services and Wales, HMSO, 1984.

The Report of the Social Service Committee on Perinatal and Neonatal Mortality, 1980 (The Short Report).

World Health Organisation Summary Report, Joint Interregional Conference on Appropriate Technology for Childbirth, 1985.

INDEX

BSP Practical Guides

All books are available through bookshops and can be purchased from NCVO Reception during office hours. In case of difficulty books can be ordered by post direct from Plymbridge Distributors Ltd, Estover Road, Plymouth PL6 7PZ (tel. 0752-705251) adding 12½% to total value of order for post and packing (minimum 45p).

For further details of any title please contact the Sales Manager, NCVO/Bedford Square Press, 26 Bedford Square, London WC1B 3HU (tel. 071-636 4066).

The Voluntary Agencies Directory 1991

The Social Activists' Bible

NCVO's directory of voluntary agencies is the standard reference work for anyone who cares about helping the community. It lists nearly 2,000 leading voluntary agencies, ranging from small, specialist self-help groups to long-established national charities. It gives concise, up-to-date descriptions of their aims and activities with details of

charitable status	local branches
volunteer participation	membership
trading activities	staffing

A list of useful addresses includes professional and public advisory bodies concerned with voluntary action; a classified index and quick reference list of acronyms and abbreviations give easy access to entries.

There is extensive coverage of groups concerned with women's issues, minority rights, self-help, community development and leisure activities, environment and conservation, campaigning and consumer affairs.

Voluntary agencies play an important part in making the world a better place to live in. This NCVO directory is the essential guide to their work.

'If you buy only one directory of voluntary agencies, buy this one and buy it every year.'   *Health Libraries Review*

'...an essential working tool.'   *Environment Now*

£10.95

The Health Directory
Compiled for the 'Thames Help' programme by Fiona Macdonald

*In association with the College of Health
and the Patients' Association*

A new edition of the former *Health Help* volume, first published by
Bedford Square Press in 1987, the 1990/91 edition lists around 1,000
organisations set up to help patients and their families with many
common (and not so common) health problems. They range from
established national bodies such as the Red Cross and the NSPCC, to
self-help groups dealing with a particular disorder.

Symbols are used to indicate when an organisation is a registered
charity, has branches or local groups, welcomes volunteers or produces
publications. The directory also includes organisations dealing with
complementary medicine, ethnic minorities and general sources of
help. The entries are listed alphabetically and in a comprehensive
index by subject order.

£6.95

The Parents' Directory
Compiled by Fiona Macdonald
Foreword by Esther Rantzen

'Whatever the problem...you only need spend a few minutes glancing through the pages of *The Parents' Directory* to see what an astonishing variety of voluntary bodies there are for parents to turn to...an excellent and comprehensive map.'   *Esther Rantzen*

The Parents Directory lists around 800 voluntary organisations which are able to give help, advice and information to parents on a wide range of topics. The information is presented in easily accessible form under the headings Education, Family Welfare, Handicap, Health and Leisure, with each entry giving details of aims and objects, contact names and telephone. Symbols are used to give additional information in the same manner as that outlined for *The Health Directory*.

£6.95

Forthcoming

The Women's Directory
Compiled by Fiona Macdonald

The Women's Directory will enable women who wish to make contact with others - whether for social, cultural, sporting, charitable, self-help or political purposes - to locate and identify suitable groups and organisations. It refers women to appropriate 'umbrella' bodies, whether voluntary, local-government-based or state funded, and gives other sources of information about women's activities, including relevant magazines and journals, publishers and bookshops. Presented in an accessible, simple-to-follow format, with symbols used to give additional information in the same manner as that outlined for *The Health Directory*.

£6.95